DYING TO SMOKE

WENDY KIRCHNER

STARR PUBLISHING
MELBOURNE, FL 32934

LIBRARY OF CONGRESS CARD NUMBER:
97-91041

ISBN 0-9659188-0-7

Printing: Printmark,Inc.
Edited by: DanaRae Pomeroy, Writer's Edge, Inc.
About the Author & 1997 family photograph by:
Chris Webre, Picture This...photography
Cover & Layout Design by: Judy Salinsky

Published in the USA by
STARR BOOKS
Starr Publishing

Dedicated to my Husband,

Harry C. Kirchner,

Never Forgotten

Lives are taken every day,
From people who just smoke away.
My father unknowing was in
A battle he could never win.

Suddenly, he began to see,
What wasn't such a mystery.
With his body now in nicotine's control,
To try and quit became impossible.

Soon he began to loose all hope,
While slipping down life's short, frayed rope.
There he fell, without a tug,
He lost his life - to America's deadliest drug.

- Kate Kirchner

Contents

Acknowledgments

My deepest gratitude to my children, Chris, Kerin and Kate, the joy of my life, for enabling me to sit at the computer, night after night, spilling their life on each page. For allowing the honesty, no matter how painful. To these fine, young adults who have taught me so much. Strength, courage and endurance. From the bottom of my heart, I love you.

My continued love and appreciation to:

The two people who gave me the wonderful gift of story telling, and the perseverance and fortitude to tell it, my mother and father. I love you and miss you. I thank you.

My brother Wayne, who has believed in me since the day I was born.

My brother Warren, for his love and encouragement to finish this book.

Claudia and Sally, my dear friends, who supported me with countless hours of listening, in my deepest, darkest hours. Who have always been there for me, and I know always will.

Gail and George, for their devoted friendship during and after Harry's illness.

My cousin Al, who gave me the self confidence to proceed with this project.

Dr. Deligdish and his staff, for their courageous battle to help Harry, allowing us to continually have hope.

Judy, a brave cancer survivor, for all your help in creating this book, designing the cover, and your friendship.

All my friends and family who had faith in me and encouraged me to finish a task which at times seemed impossible.

And, to all of you who become believers...Who tackle the difficult challenge of quitting smoking, and win...

God bless you all....

Foreword

Cigarettes will kill approximately 155,000 people this year. In the United States alone, lung cancer will take that many lives. It is the leading fatal cancer in both men and women.

Lung cancer has risen rapidly because of the spread of cigarette smoking in developing countries. An increasing degree of cancer has been clearly observed over the past few decades, due in part to improved cancer testing, the increase of life expectancy, and also, due to the increase of tobacco smokers.

The people who die from this demeaning disease are not the only victims. Cancer tears families apart and leaves the survivors to sort through the pieces. Vivid memories of cancer's destruction are hard to forget. Thousands of people have lived this nightmare already, or are about to. One account, taken from such a substantial number of unfortunate sufferers may seem insignificant. But it isn't, when cancer's prey is someone close to your heart.

This is one family's story. Our story. Our struggle with lung cancer, diagnosed in my husband Harry, the father of our three children. Of how he continued to smoke, despite valiant efforts to try and save him. Of our battle against nicotine and its invincible hold.

Of how it won.

It took a great deal of courage and pain, to put our family's tragedy on paper for all to see. However, it was important to me that Harry not become just another statistic. He was a good husband and father, which gave his life significant meaning.

Unfortunately, Harry did not believe tobacco was harmful. He denied all the facts and statistics, thought they were greatly exaggerated. Now that the addictive effects of tar and nicotine are more widely known, however, it is much clearer to me why Harry was so completely and thoroughly hooked. Until quite recently, an abundance of misleading information had been distributed to the general public by the heads of the tobacco companies. (More on that in the chapter Why Quit). Thank goodness these companies are now being held accountable for their actions and, hopefully, will eventually be brought to justice.

Cigarettes took him away from us. Our knowledge and awareness of that cannot bring Harry back. Our only redemption can be to change people's ideas and beliefs; to convince them that cigarettes and/or other forms of tobacco, are deadly weapons.

Don't allow yourself or your loved one to become another lung cancer statistic. It is the one form of cancer that is preventable!

But you must stop smoking, now.

Harry paid the ultimate price for those costly cigarettes. He paid with his life.

Chapter 1

"Till death do you part." For years, married couples have uttered those words, unconsciously accepting their meaning. If the marriage is lucky enough to defy the odds, one does expect to care for each other in the twilight years. But when you are both thirty seven, working diligently and raising three very lively children, "till death do you part," doesn't enter the mind much. Life is too busy being lived, to think of death.

Until the someone you love announces one day, "I have cancer." Suddenly, the world in which you live, stops abruptly. A whirlwind of doctors, hospitals, and medical lingo spins you totally out of control. Almost immediately, you learn what you must do. Hold each other tight, take each day as it comes,and hang on.

It was Feb. 28,1991, my older brother's birthday. I had just asked myself if I had remembered to mail his card. But this day would become one that we would all remember, for a much different reason. In one split second, our family priorities would do a handstand.

I answered the phone at work, something I did dozens of times a day. It was my husband's voice on the other end, but Harry sounded strange. Very quiet and subdued. He asked me to come home. Oddly, I didn't know he was getting his test results back from his doctor's visit that day. He hadn't mentioned it. Therefore, I had no idea what was going on.

I asked him several times, but he wouldn't say what was wrong. My father was there and Harry didn't want to talk in front of him. I could feel my heart begin to race. Not wanting to wait to relieve my heart wrenching pains of curiosity, I asked him to go to our bedroom phone.

Suddenly, the deep silence stopped. Harry had begun to cry. I was startled beyond belief. "What's the matter, Harry?" I shouted.

After what seemed like an eternity, he blurted it out. "*I have lung cancer*!"

I honestly didn't think I had heard him right. How in the world does a *blood doctor* find lung cancer? I was so confused. I know I asked him several times, how did the doctor know, how could he be sure? My repetition seems so cruel now. I put Harry on hold and went into the bank lunchroom. I grabbed the phone and began to weep. No one was saying a word. There were just sobs, between two people who should have been in each other's arms, and yet, had to settle for the warmth of each other's voice.

I told him I would be right home.

I reflect back on that drive. It was only seven miles, and yet, there were *miles and miles* of thoughts crammed into my head. I had the feeling of complete helplessness. I didn't know what to say or do.

When I got in the door, my father was sitting in the den, on the couch, totally unaware. I hurried past him, barely giving him a hello, went into our bedroom and closed the door. Harry was sitting on the edge of the bed, facing the window, just gazing out, alone. It is a picture that will remain in my mind forever.

We held each other for a long time. I had been so worried about what to say, but words weren't really necessary. After the long stretch of silence, Harry said, "You know, I'm sitting here thinking that you have it harder than I do. I have to fight for my life. But if I don't make it, you have the kids...You have three kids to raise."

It was the only time he ever alluded to the thought he might die. I told him not to think that way – that he could beat this. That he was so young. I honestly believe, once that thought left his mind that day, he never let it back in. Harry *believed* he was going to live.

We sat and talked quietly for the best part of an hour. Suddenly, our thirteen year old son, Chris, burst into the room, home from school, ready to share his day. I'm certain he could tell there was something quite different about *this one.* Harry stood up, walked over to him, and softly told him that he had lung cancer. He then put his arms around his son and hugged him.

This must have been overwhelming for Chris. Harry was not usually a demonstrative type of father. Chris just stood there, his arms dangling at his sides, speechless. I related to his obvious feeling of complete helplessness. Here he was, just dropping in to say hello, and I'm sure he got more than he expected. Harry told him not to worry, that he was going to have whatever kind of treatment was necessary and he was going to be all right. Chris nodded his head and left.

My poor father was still sitting on the couch, undoubtedly wondering why he was being ignored. I called him into the room and told him about the cancer. He went up to Harry and hugged him. With firmness and fortitude, he said, "They've come a long way, with all kinds of new treatments today. I'm sure they can help you, Harry. You're such a young man." He hugged me also, and told me to count on his help, whenever it was needed. He left, respecting our need for privacy.

A short while later we called Harry's parents, Peggy and Harry Sr., in New York. How awful for them to get such devastating news, and be so far away. We all cried uncontrollably. They hung up, saying they would call back when they were able to talk.

Everything changed drastically that day. Life, as the Kirchners knew it, would never be the same.

The following day at work, things were strange. It was an uncomfortable situation. No one knew what to say. I had no idea just how used to that reaction I would have to get.

I felt very alone.

On Wednesday, March 6th, Harry and I had an appointment to meet with Dr. Deligdish, together. He was an *oncologist* and *hematologist,* a doctor specializing in cancer and diseases of the blood. It now made sense, how this blood doctor knew he had cancer.

Waiting in the lobby was enlightening. There was no one under sixty. Of course, there are lots of young people with cancer, but there were none in the room that day, or any other day for that matter. We certainly stood out.

Dr. Deligdish was unlike any doctor I had ever seen. His hair was long and disheveled. He was about 5'7" and extremely thin. He appeared to be about our age. That alone was shocking. I searched in his long, slender face for some reassurance, but found none. He was professional, but quite clinical. I guess I wanted Dr. Deligdish to tell us it was all going to be O.K. Instead, here was a man who knew his business, knew the odds, and knew it was better to be direct, rather than condescending.

I had no idea how wrong my perception was. Not only would this man become a partner in the fight against Harry's cancer, but he would help me find the strength to fight that battle as well.

I don't remember all the doctor said that day. Only bits and pieces come back to me. I was too overwhelmed by this young, hip, M.D., and too busy watching Harry's reactions, to really listen to what he was saying. He did recommend surgery. He explained that many lung cancers are not operable. In Harry's case, though, because of his young age, he was sure a surgeon would agree it was a necessary option.

Dr. Deligdish did not feel the cancer had spread yet. It was then I began to learn the depth of my ignorance on the subject. There are several types of cancer. Previously, I had thought, when you have cancer, you have cancer. Wrong. Also, as strange as it may seem, there are some cancers that are better to have than others. Some are slow growing, while others grow quite rapidly. Harry, unfortunately, was not one of the "lucky" ones. Lung cancer is usually a type that will *metastasize*, or spread. Early detection does help. But in Harry's case, it became clear later on, his cancer had been spreading for a long time.

The doctor asked if we had any questions. Harry did not. He was very quiet. I wanted to know about the operation and what would be involved. Treatment would start with radiation, which would help to shrink the tumor. Surgery would follow, to remove the remaining tumor and any other cancer cells found. Because of the cancer's presence, one third of the lung, part of the chest wall, and three or four ribs would have to be removed. *Unbelievable*.

Dr. Deligdish then stated that if Harry remained in *remission,* or cancer free, for five years, his chance of survival was good. Lung cancer, however, usually reoccurs within a year. If that happened, a new treatment plan would have to be decided upon at that time.

He recommended that we go to the social security office to apply for benefits. Harry qualified for disability, having such a serious disease as lung cancer.

I walked outside, alone, while Harry stayed a few minutes to give a blood sample, one of hundreds that would be taken, in the upcoming months.

My head was spinning. This couldn't possibly be happening to us. I wanted to wake up from this horrid nightmare. I know I desperately wanted to keep things *normal.* Since cancer had now taken over every aspect of our lives, I had no idea how difficult that would be.

We drove to the Social Security office in almost complete silence, followed by two grueling hours of questions and paperwork. One particularly painful moment remains forever in my mind. The social security clerk asked Harry if he was terminal. Point blank. Just like that. What else could he answer, but that he didn't know? It was heart wrenching to witness.

On the way home, Harry broke the silence. "Do you want to know what the kind nurse told me today in the doctor's office? She said she believes things like this happen for a reason. To wake you up, make you appreciate life and the ones you love more. Wasn't that really a wonderful thing for her to say?"

Yes, Harry, it truly was.

Chapter 2

Harry and I were married March 20,1976. The *Bicentennial Year*. That really is how I remember! We were both twenty three. We'd worked together, as tellers in a bank, for a year before we started dating, and wound up together at the infamous office Christmas party. Harry was the only man I'd ever dated that smoked. Although it was a deep concern of mine, once we became engaged, he promised me he would quit. I believed him.

There was something mysterious about Harry. He always kept you guessing, as to what was on his mind and what made him tick. Aside from his good looks, thick, dark hair and sky blue eyes, it was his great sense of humor that initiated my attraction. Harry could be hilariously funny, but in a very quiet, discreet way. He was never the life of a party. Harry was usually in the corner somewhere, keeping whoever was nearby in stitches. Humor has always been a prerequisite of mine. I make it a point not to take life too seriously and to find the humor in most situations. The banter is what started our friendship and the banter is what turned the friendship into something more.

Little did I know, however, just how complex this man really was. The laughter disguised a very intelligent, but reclusive young man who just didn't let people in...*Private.* His thoughts and feelings were his and his alone.

I fought this trait of him, our entire married life. Every once in a while, a really profound thought would emerge, one that made you realize Harry really did think things through. But that was a rare and unique moment.

Our son, Christopher Patrick Kirchner was born July 16,1977, a short sixteen months after our marriage. We were inexperienced but proud parents, and we were twenty four. My entire pregnancy, Harry assured me he would quit smoking before the baby came. He promised. Even though he had given his oath before we were married, I still believed him. I just knew he wouldn't want to smoke around our new baby.

During my pregnancy, there was a television commercial in which a handsome, wise, father and his adorable, blond, blue-eyed son were resting together, leaned up against a tree. The father pulled out a cigarette pack and began to light one up. The little boy looked up at his father and asked, "Why do you smoke, Daddy? Isn't it bad for you?" Suddenly, the father looked at his young son, crushed the box and threw the cigarettes over his shoulder.

I just knew Harry would feel the same way.

When our new pride and joy came home, the cigarettes came, too. Harry never stopped, not even for a day. I begged. I pleaded. I nagged. Nothing worked. Quite a few times, I caught him feeding the baby his bottle with a cigarette hanging from his mouth. I had a fit!

I was so hurt. Harry had not kept his promise.

I didn't realize it then, but the nicotine had already taken hold of Harry and wouldn't let go.

Three years later, on July 28, 1980, Kerin Margaret Kirchner, our beautiful baby daughter, arrived. Again, I begged Harry to quit smoking, but it never happened.

We had a small, two bedroom apartment, and the two kids shared a room. Money was tight, very tight. I had stopped working, so Harry began to work two jobs.

In the meantime, my parents, retired and moved to Florida,

and I missed them terribly.

We were living a stressful existence in cramped quarters.

In 1981, with the help of my parents and my brother, Wayne, we scraped up a down payment for a small, "handyman special" home in Bay Shore, Long Island. We were now the proud owners of one dog, two kids, and a thirty year mortgage! All at the ripe age of twenty seven.

The following year, my mother passed away suddenly, in her sleep, of a brain hemorrhage. She was only sixty four. This was the first person close to me to die. I had an extremely hard time dealing with her death and could barely function. My children were one and four, and needed me. I couldn't comprehend how life still went on. People got up, went to work, came home, ate dinner. The sun still rose and set each day. *No one else's life* seemed to change drastically, except my own. Why should this happen to *my mother?* Life was not fair. I was sad, angry, depressed.

I digress for a reason. It was my mother's death that paved the way for me to become a stronger person. I learned how to cope with my bereavement, and came to realize all my feelings were normal. *My mother's death taught me about life.*

On May 20, 1983, another lovely daughter, Kathryn Margaret Kirchner arrived. Purely unexpected, but loved all the more. With each child's birth, I reminded Harry how much money we could save, if he would just quit smoking. It could help pay for diapers, formula, and that thirty year mortgage. Each time, he would mumble, tell me how he hated to be nagged, and how much he loved to smoke. I was discouraged, but truthfully dismissed all serious thoughts about it. After all, I knew there was plenty of time to convince him to quit. We were only thirty.

In September, 1984, we moved to a bigger home, ten miles down the road, in a quaint old town called Oakdale. This house also needed work, but Harry and I could handle it. We had both gotten rather handy and creative. Necessity truly is the mother of invention.

A new house and three wonderful, healthy children. Life was great. And we were only thirty three.

In January of 1985, a good friend of ours, Gary Genari, died of lung cancer. He was thirty eight, a smoker, who had quit five years before. Gary died just a short nine months after being diagnosed. Harry and I had worked with his wife, Janice, when we were tellers. Gary was a sergeant in the local police department. Over the years, we'd kept in touch, and eventually bought homes around the corner from each other. Gary and Janice had twin girls, seven years old at the time. This family had everything in the world going for them. It was such a tragedy.

Gary's death really hit home for me. I knew this could be Harry. I couldn't imagine living through such an ordeal. Janice, a young widow, those poor little girls, having to grow up without a father. It was more than I could bare to even think about.

I begged Harry to quit. I cried. We began to fight about it. I couldn't understand how he could witness Gary's death from this awful disease, leaving his family behind, and not be affected by it all. I purchased every item on the market that promised to help people quit smoking. Gum, cassette tapes, filters for the end of the cigarettes. Harry used the filters, threw them away, and smoked even more. Nothing worked. Harry was truly hooked.

Whenever I brought up my fear of his becoming ill, his perpetual comment was, "We all have to die of something, someday." Do people who smoke really believe this? It makes no sense to me.

I waged war against those cigarettes. They were winning.

In February of 1987, during a visit with my father in Florida, we decided to move south. Long Island had become so crowded and expensive, we were both ready for a change. We eagerly put money down on a lot in Melbourne, Florida. Within six months, we packed up the house, the dog, and the kids. We had no jobs, so certainly we were taking a chance. But risk-taking is for the young, and that we were. We were only thirty four.

On our journey to Melbourne, we passed a group of log cabin models along the highway in North Carolina. Exhausted from the long ride, we decided to stop and take a look. Harry and I were delightfully surprised. We loved those cabins. We gathered all the literature we could. We made plans to purchase a kit, later on, once things had settled down from our move.

Our goal was to build one of these cabins on a lake, to use as a family summer home. We had both become so handy, with our fixer-up homes, we knew we were up to the task. It would be both adventurous and enjoyable.

A new home in Florida. A summer cabin on a lake. These were our hopes and dreams. We had no idea that before very long, all our hopes and dreams would go *up in smoke*.

Chapter 3

Studies have shown that stress can sometimes be an important factor in the development of cancer growth. I am convinced that during this period of time, when Harry was looking for work, his cancer began.

It took over six months for Harry to find a suitable job. He worked odd jobs, digging ditches, stacking cookies, moving office furniture, anything to bring in some cash. While waiting for his big break, he was depressed and often angry. He smoked more than ever. I know he never expected it to take so long to find work. None of us did.

We fought over the fact that money was extremely tight, yet he still found extra to buy those cigarettes. How could he possibly justify such an extravagant expense? Still, the more stressful things became, the more he smoked.

In April of 1988, Harry finally landed a job as a branch manager with a local savings & loan. It was not the dream job he was looking or hoping for, but it would do for a while. We now had medical benefits and a steady paycheck. Life was good again. Besides, there was lots of time ahead for those hopes and dreams. We were only thirty five.

Our days were busy. I had a part-time job, Harry was employed and the kids' assorted sports, plays and piano lessons, kept us content and occupied.

In 1989, the savings & loan crisis was at its peak. Harry was beginning to worry he might lose his job. I dreaded even the thought of that possibility and secretly hoped he was just being overly cautious. In November of 1990, however, our worst fear became reality. Harry was notified he would be laid off the following January.

When he called me at work, with the dreadful news, I thought my world had come tumbling down. There was a mortgage, a car payment, and three kids to feed. How were the bills going to be paid? We both knew the chances of him obtaining another bank job were nil. With the savings crisis, banks weren't hiring. He'd been out of work before and the economy was even worse now. I tried to be optimistic and encouraging, but it was difficult. Harry had to be scared to death as well, but didn't dare discuss it with me. We were both trying to protect each other from the inevitable distress.

Fortunately, I had gone full-time at my bank job a few months before. I hadn't really wanted to, as I knew how hectic it would be, but Harry and I agreed that I would take the available position, temporarily. Just until he landed a new job that was secure. It turned out to be a critical decision.

Harry was tense and had a real short fuse with all of us. He began to paint the house, partly because it needed it, mostly because he needed something to do. Shortly after he started, he stopped. He complained that his shoulder hurt, probably from the back and forth strokes of the brush. At the time, it made sense. Now, however, I question my reasoning. After all, Harry was only thirty seven years old. With the many repairs and such he'd done in the past, why should a little painting bother his shoulder — to that extent? I know I was convinced he was depressed. And depression can cause all kinds of ailments. I was sure all his symptoms would go away once he found a job.

The pain continued. Harry would lay awake night after night, with a heating pad on his shoulder, and have me rub ointment on the aching joint. This was completely out of character for Harry. He'd never complained of aches or pains before and he *never* took sick time from work. Strange as it may seem, Harry was probably one of the healthiest individuals I'd ever known.

Late November, 1990, Harry began to see a chiropractor. Previously, he had questioned their usefulness, but alas, he now found himself at the mercy of one. Three times a week, he was put on all kinds of machines, and given several electrode treatments. At the end of six weeks, the doctor asked Harry if he was feeling any relief. Since he was not, the chiropractor recommended he see a medical doctor. But Christmas was right around the corner, we had a lot of shopping to do and many more bills to pay.

Christmas of 1990 was not very merry. Neither Harry, Chris, nor I were feeling very good. I had bronchitis, which robbed me of my usual energy. Chris caught it from me, so we certainly were a house full of sick people. But Kerin and Kate were ten and seven at the time, so we put up a good front and celebrated as best we could.

In January, Harry went to the local walk-in clinic. Their diagnosis was simple. A pulled muscle in his shoulder. He was given an anti-inflammatory drug and told to come back in a week, if he didn't feel better. Harry didn't feel much better; he went back, and was given a stronger dosage.

When I look back upon how I felt during this time, it's difficult to admit my indifference. I really believed this was all brought on by unhappiness and stress. I saw a depressed man who was soon going to be out of work and had not yet found another job. Four people were depending on him for the roof over their head and severance pay only lasts so long. Each evening, I would massage his shoulder and tell him that he would feel better once he got a job.

Hang in there, Harry. You'll get a job.

January 18th was Harry's last day at work. One of his tellers called me and told me they all came in wearing black that day. His employees were all upset about his lay-off. I was deeply grateful and moved by her phone call. Once we hung up, I cried my eyes out. I could only wonder what was to become of us. Would we have to sell the house? Move? I couldn't comprehend why such a terrible thing was happening to us. I had no idea of the *real nightmare* we were about to enter.

When the stronger dosage of muscle relaxer still didn't relieve the pain in Harry's shoulder, the doctor recommended he be seen by an Internist. The new doctor ran a series of tests, including a chest x-ray, which were *all* inconclusive. It was this doctor, however, who told Harry, "I don't know what you have, but whatever it is, don't worry, it's not life threatening." Later on, when I had to be in touch with this man, he told me how completely shocked he was by Harry's diagnosis. He claimed Harry was one of the healthiest looking, seriously ill, patients he had ever seen.

A week before Harry's next appointment, his parents came to visit. They came bearing gifts, as always; Harry's was a carton of cigarettes. They knew this made me unhappy, but Peggy glanced over at me and explained, "Well, he's going to buy them anyway." She was right.

One evening, after dinner, Peggy expressed her concerns to me about Harry's medical condition. She couldn't understand how he could have this shoulder pain for such a long time. I know I was trying to minimize her worry, but I explained that Harry was not a happy man, knowing he was going to be out of work. I honestly believed my words. I realize now, I should have paid closer attention.

Harry was referred to Dr. Craig Deligdish, board certified hematologist and oncologist. Harry told me he was going to a blood doctor. He never mentioned the oncologist part. I don't know whether this was intentional or not.

After a thorough physical and several blood tests, Dr. Deligdish ordered a *CAT scan,* an x-ray procedure that uses a computer to produce a detailed picture of a section of the body. I wasn't aware of this at the time, but doctors do not order this type of test at random. They are quite expensive, ($800-$900), so the insurance companies insist that the doctor be almost certain that *something* is there, which doesn't belong there. However, when you're naive about the procedures of the medical world, as we certainly were, there's an awful lot to learn.

Harry's results from his CAT-scan came back and he was scheduled for a consultation on the infamous February 28th. He went, of course. Unfortunately, this was the one appointment he shouldn't have gone to alone.

Chapter 4

A few weeks after Harry and I met with Dr. Deligdish, Harry decided to get a second opinion. He and his parents thought it would be best for him to be seen at *Memorial Sloan-Kettering Institute,* in New York. Since his parents lived nearby, on Long Island, they could take him back and forth to the hospital. As much as I hated to see him go away, I completely agreed with his decision. *Sloan-Kettering* was a reputable cancer hospital, and a second opinion was definitely necessary with such a serious illness as lung cancer.

We agreed, if he should decide to be operated on up there, I would fly up and be with him. My Dad would stay with the kids. It was all set.

Harry called Dr. Deligdish's office, explained what he wanted to do, and requested a copy of his medical files. They were both accommodating and understanding, and quickly got his transcripts together for him.

The night before he was to leave, two girlfriends of mine came over with a thoughtful "basket of cheer" for Harry, filled with all kinds of handy paraphernalia for him to take to New York. Decks of cards, crossword puzzle books, gum and life-savers were just a few of the assorted items. Their kind thoughts and gestures were greatly appreciated.

Since we didn't have much family around us, (other than my father, of course), our kind and caring friends helped fill the void.

On March 15th, I took Harry to the airport. We hugged for a long time and said our goodbyes. I was so sad. I really didn't want him to go. This was the first time in our marriage he'd gone away without me. I'd taken a few vacations to Florida, with the kids, to visit my Dad, leaving Harry in New York, but it had never been the other way around. Never before had I taken care of the kids and the house, by myself. As much as I am a very independent woman in many ways, I relied on Harry for his strength and calmness, and most of all, his love and support.

Harry's parents met him at LaGuardia Airport and they drove directly to *Sloan-Kettering.* The place must have been enormous, quite a change from the warmth of Dr. Deligdish's small, informal office. After a lengthy wait, Harry was eventually seen by an Indian doctor. He examined him for a few minutes, more or less listened to his heart and pulse. Harry wanted to know what was next. The doctor explained he would have to look over the medical reports and findings and get back to him with his diagnosis. He excused himself and that was that.

Harry and his parents left for home. Three or four days later, Harry called *Sloan*, as he hadn't heard anything. The doctor still hadn't looked at his charts.

March 20th was our fifteenth wedding anniversary. We'd spent every anniversary together before this, and it was so lonely and strange to be apart. We talked on the phone for a while, trying to fill the void, but it was not the same. Two of my aunts sent us each the same anniversary card which I thought was so kind.

Finally, after two more days, Harry was called back in. The doctor's findings were in agreement with Dr. Deligdish's, in that there was a tumor on the lung. But, his recommendation for treatment was quite different. Massive dosages of chemotherapy for four to five weeks, then wait and see how the cancer responded. No surgery was recommended. In his medical opinion, surgery wouldn't help. When Harry phoned me with the results, I was quite confused. I didn't know what to think. Why would this doctor's opinion contrast with Dr. Deligdish's to such a degree?

I came to my own conclusions later on. I truly believe *Sloan-Kettering* felt that Harry's case was hopeless. They must have felt there was no point in operating, if the chance of eradicating the cancer was so slim.

Nevertheless, Harry needed time to consider all his options. Two days later, he phoned me. His tone was different. He told me he wanted to come home. He wanted to be back with his wife and kids and that he'd decided to be treated by Dr. Deligdish and his wonderful, kind and supportive staff. I was thrilled, of course. I'd hoped he would come to that decision, but it had to come from Harry, and it did.

When Harry called Deligdish's office, to let them know he was coming back, the nurse was both compassionate and understanding. "Oh, Harry. I'm so glad you're coming back to us. We'll take good care of you."

The *American Cancer Society* states, "Education, reassurance and love are all necessary for the complete care of the cancer patient." At Dr. Deligdish's office, Harry was treated with all of those. He was not just a number. He was a human being. I witnessed Dr. Deligdish's attempt to help Harry with every possible treatment available. And for that, I am forever grateful.

Chapter 5

Before Harry left for New York, he'd asked me not to tell anyone (other than the few people that already knew) that he had lung cancer. I really didn't agree, or understand, but respected his wishes.

While he was away however, I realized we both needed all the love and support from family and friends we could get. I knew people would find out sooner or later and cancer was certainly nothing to be ashamed of. I think Harry just did not want anyone's pity.

A few days before Harry came home, I ran into a neighbor from the next street, Glen. Harry had struck up a 'big-brother' type of relationship with the younger man, who was married with a baby boy. Both men enjoyed helping each other with yard work and had been known to share a beer...or two! Glen stared in amazement, as I told him about Harry's illness. His father was dying of cancer at the time, which I knew, but of course he didn't mention it. He just wanted to know how he could help. He said he would stop by when Harry got back.

I also called another friend of Harry's, George, who, along with his wife, Gail, had been good friends to both of us. Because of our busy schedules, we hadn't been in touch in a while, but I knew George would be a tremendous help. He was a big, burly, jovial sort of guy, the kind that always had a joke or allowed himself to be the butt of one. I knew this was the kind of friend Harry needed back in his life.

Once back from New York, Harry met with Dr. Deligdish and his treatment plan was set up. He would start with four weeks of radiation, which would help shrink the tumor, making the surgery, scheduled for May 7th, easier and less complicated.

I ran into Glen again, at the local grocery store, and mentioned that Harry was back. He told me he was off that day and he might stop by. Luckily, I had confessed to Harry I had not kept my promise of silence. I know he understood, but he just shook his head and sighed.

Glen came over with two large bottles of beer. We all sat in the den and started small talk. To my and Glen's great surprise, Harry turned down the offer of the beer. "I'm trying to live healthier now," was all he said. It was obvious Glen didn't know how to respond. That beer guzzling bond was gone. The mood changed, as Glen and I struggled to keep the conversation going.

But Harry clearly didn't want to be there. He didn't want to drink beer, or sit and talk, certainly not about cancer. Harry didn't want people to treat him differently and yet, that was impossible. He was different, things were different. There was *not a thing* anyone could do about that.

Harry's first weekend home, my brother Warren, arrived from Colorado, with his new girlfriend. He hadn't been in town for a year and had called to say he wanted to come by for a visit. It was later I learned his girlfriend had told him how serious lung cancer was and that he'd better get to Florida to help his sister and visit with his extremely ill brother-in-law.

We had a wonderful visit. Although Harry was relatively quiet and rested a lot, things were light, airy and fun. They stayed five days. The night before they were leaving, April 9th, they brought in an ice cream cake, to celebrate Harry's birthday, a day early. He would be thirty eight.

I was really glad they'd come. It enabled us to "get away from it all", for a short while.

Harry spent his thirty eighth birthday receiving his first radiation treatment. He joked with the technicians, telling them the least they could do was give him that treatment free. When he arrived home, he held a T-shirt in his hand. He smirked as he opened it to reveal the message. "*My Magnetic Personality came from Holmes Regional Hospital. M R I.*" I tried to hide the fact that I was startled. Harry seemed to think it was funny, so I played along. I really didn't get it though. Harry's cancer was a life and death situation. Who would want to wear a T-shirt announcing one is undergoing radiation? In time, though, it began to make some sense. After all, chemotherapy, radiation, cancer. It's nothing to hide or be ashamed of. Anyone who is fighting the battle of cancer, *in any way*, becomes a stronger, better person. They certainly deserve our love and respect. May they all proudly wear their T-shirts.

Harry had radiation treatments three times a week. Almost immediately, I noticed a decrease in his appetite. The radiation didn't make him nauseous, but it greatly reduced his desire to eat. He also became quite tired. Whereas Harry usually had quite a lot of constructive energy, I found him to be somewhat lethargic. Giving himself an emotionally encouraging boost, he would say, over and over, "At least it's not chemo." He was so happy not to have to deal with that. Consequently, he put up with the radiation's side effects. In four weeks, he lost about fifteen pounds. At 5'9", and with his beginning weight of 165, he didn't need to lose any weight. But, even though he may have been a little thinner, he still looked pretty good, all things considered.

While Harry was driving himself to his treatments, I went to work. I tried desperately to keep everything routine in our home. I told the kids that Daddy had cancer, and that some people die from it, but Daddy was young, was going to have surgery, and was going to be all right.

The girls seemed to leave it up to me, to fill them in on whatever was going on. I told them only what I felt they needed to know. After all, at seven and ten, life was simple and pure. I wanted to protect them from all the scary, unknown feelings I was experiencing. I acted pretty "normal", I think.

Chris, however, *wanted to know.* He was born with that inquisitive mind that questioned everything. Why wouldn't he want to know what was going on with his father's life? At age thirteen, I knew he was old enough to deal with the facts. I was always completely honest. I felt I owed him that. Although Chris was still a "kid" in every way, there was a lot of maturity behind that curious mind.

Slowly, over time, communication between Harry and I got worse, instead of better. Harry spent a lot more time "resting" in our room. I would plead with him, over and over, "Talk to me, tell me what you're feeling." He never talked about the cancer. Ever. That subject was taboo. He would have been forced to reach in and pull out emotions he wasn't comfortable sharing, with me, or anyone else. It was the early stages of complete denial. I tried to make him understand that even though he was the one with the cancer, because I was his wife and because I loved him, — we were in this together. I tried desperately to get him to open up, but I never had much success.

Some things would not change.

May 7th was coming quickly. The week before the scheduled operation, Harry and I met with the two assigned surgeons, at their office. Harry had been given a cardiogram and "scored" very high. Better than his own, Dr. Palmer had said.

Dr. Battaglini did most of the talking. He was a very calm, soft-spoken man, who made us both feel quite at ease, as he explained all that was going to take place.

The operation was called a *lobectomy*, and involved removing either a part or all of a lobe from a lung. They would also have to remove three or four back ribs, in order to remove the tumor. It had entwined itself into them, therefore making it necessary to take them out, and any more cancer cells or tumors with them. He explained this would cause Harry's left shoulder to have a slight droop, but to the average person would be barely noticeable. *Unbelievable*. He also stated they would check wherever possible for any other cancer cells, and if found, remove them. If you left even one, it would most likely *metastasize* and form a new tumor somewhere else.

It was his belief, however, that the cancer was confined to the one area, in the shoulder. The CAT scan had not revealed any other tumors and certainly that was a good sign. Dr. Battaglini also made the statement, like Dr. Deligdish, that if Harry remained cancer free, after surgery, for five years, he would have a good chance of staying in remission, and surviving.

As much as I'm certain all doctors want to be positive and encouraging, whenever possible, I still believe they all felt, at that point, Harry Kirchner had pretty good odds.

There was hope.

28. . . dying to smoke

Chapter 6

May 7th arrived, and we were ready. Harry's parents were planning to come down after his surgery. My father would stay at my house and help with the house and kids, until Harry's folks arrived.

Harry and I got to the hospital at 6:30 in the morning for last minute blood tests and procedures. His operation was scheduled for 10:00 a.m. and would take approximately three hours. About nine o'clock, they wheeled him up to his room to wait. His mood was somewhat somber, but I tried to make small talk just the same. We watched television, off and on. Watched as the rest of the world went on with their lives, while ours stood still.

A nurse came in and announced there's been an emergency open heart surgery; Harry's appointed time was pushed forward. His operation would be rescheduled for sometime later in the day. What a cruel twist of fate. Harry moaned, but there was nothing anyone could do. They would come for him probably around lunch time.

She asked if anyone had explained what to expect after the surgery, explaining it would be less frightening if we knew up front. We agreed and stated we really didn't know, so she began.

When Harry came out of the recovery room, he would be connected to several tubes, two from his lungs, and a drainage tube coming out of his side. He'd be receiving blood, antibiotics, and glucose. He would also be receiving nourishment through a feeding tube, as it would be a while before he could eat whole food. He would be catheterized and hooked up to a respirator, until his one good lung functioned on its own. He would also be connected to a "pain button," containing morphine, which he could press whenever necessary. It would be impossible to overdose, however, as it is set up to only administer so many cc's per minute. *Pretty amazing...Pretty overwhelming.*

The nurse asked if we had any questions. We did not. I'm sure we both had heard all we could handle at that point. She left and we both sat there, silent for a few minutes. Suddenly, Harry began to cry. I was stunned, at first, but quickly leaned over the bed and held him in my arms. He sobbed uncontrollably. I kept telling him he would be all right. I softly stroked his hair and face until he composed himself.

He shook his head, almost in disbelief that he could behave in such a manner. Harry, the quiet, reserved man who was always in control. But for heaven's sake, why couldn't he give himself a break? He never said a word, but it appeared that, suddenly, reality had set in. This operation was serious business. It was life and death.

Once again, I could only imagine what he was thinking at that point.

A short while later, the anesthesiologist came in. He introduced himself and described the procedures, which would be used during the operation to keep Harry asleep. He then asked Harry if he would like a pill that would help "relax" him, while he waited. He understood that the delay must be unnerving and stressful. Harry didn't hesitate for a second and quickly swallowed the pill. The kind, young man then shook both our hands and left.

It was almost noon, when I realized I'd better call my father, to let him know the surgery was postponed. I went down the hall and was instructed to use a phone in a waiting room for local calls. I called my father and told him what was happening. I also told him Harry's mother would probably be calling, anxiously wanting to know what was happening. I wanted him to be sure and let her know it would still be some time yet.

I guess I should have thought to tell him to call her, but I didn't. It was not an intentional oversight. I honestly thought she would automatically call my father, figuring he would be the "central point" to whom I would report.

I hurried back to Harry. The poor guy must have been starving. He hadn't been allowed any food or water since midnight the night before. It was lunch time and he still hadn't been taken to surgery. I continued to talk to him, reassuring him it would be any time.

The minutes seemed like hours. Finally, at 12:45 p.m., an orderly came in, checked Harry's wristband and announced they were ready for him now. I kissed Harry good-bye, hugged him with all my might and told him I loved him.

"I love you too," he said with a long sigh and the best smile he could manage. I listened to the gurney's squeaky wheels as they rolled him away. I watched them take my husband down the long, tranquil hallway and enter the closed doors.

People say that the loved ones of cancer patients have it every bit as difficult or if not harder than, the patient. Although I wasn't going to be under the knife that day, it might as well have been me. To witness someone you love undergo such hurt and anguish is a pain that is indescribable. I truly was suffering, too.

I walked down to the waiting room and sat. Harry's waiting was over, but mine had just begun.

One thing is certain. The Harry they wheeled back later on was not the same man who'd gone into surgery.

The real Harry Kirchner was put to sleep that day, and never woke up.

32. . . dying to smoke

Chapter 7

I must have been sitting in the waiting room for two hours or so, when my girlfriend, Gail, George's wife, came in. She'd called my father to ask how Harry had done in surgery. He'd told her about the delay, and that I was alone, so she came up to keep me company. She truly was God-sent. I was so happy to see her!

Gail noticed I was shaking. Stupidly, I had worn shorts to the hospital, forgetting how cold hospitals can be. As a result of my bare legs and frayed nerves, I trembled like a leaf. Gail kept huddling next to me, not only to keep me warm, but to comfort me as well. We chatted occasionally, but I was really concentrating on my watch and wondering why it was taking so long. I didn't know that, even though they had taken Harry at almost one o'clock, he'd been kept in a holding room for a while. The actual surgery didn't start until after two.

At four o'clock, a nurse came in, looking for me. I jumped right up, but she only wanted to report that Harry was doing fine and the surgery was still going on. I sat back down. Again, we waited. Five o'clock passed, five thirty, then six. I *knew* something had to be wrong. Why was it taking so long? Poor Gail couldn't possibly have known what to say or do.

It was almost seven o'clock when Dr. Palmer appeared at the end of the hallway. He made eye contact with me and I studied his expression. He wasn't smiling. I felt like I was living in some bad soap opera episode. The kind where the doctor has bad news for the poor, unfortunate patient's family and he would always have that same look on his face. Somber, stern, no smile. I knew that look of gloom. My knees begin to quiver. I could do nothing but wait for him to approach me.

"Hi, Mrs. Kirchner. Let's go to the conference room, where we can have some privacy."

I glanced over at Gail, then responded, "Is it all right if my sister comes along?" I don't know why I lied to him at that point, as I'm sure it would have been fine for Gail to come, regardless of who she was. But I felt as though I were going to collapse and I knew I really needed her there. He agreed and turned to walk down the hall. We followed. No one said a word.

Once inside the small room, filled with neatly placed, milky-white tables and chairs, we all took a seat. Dr. Palmer scanned the room. "Where are Harry's parents? He *does* have parents, doesn't he?" he asked.

"They're not here. They live in New York, and have decided not to come until after he's home from the hospital," I told him.

The doctor looked quite puzzled. "Don't they realize *how serious* this is?" Again I explained that they were coming later on.

Dr. Palmer described the surgical procedure in detail, assuring me Harry was safe in the recovery room. He paused before continuing. "Harry pulled through the surgery fine, Mrs. Kirchner, but I'm afraid I don't have very good news for you." Gail took my hand. "Truthfully, if he had been an older man, we would have closed him right up. But because of his age and having a wife and three young children, we were determined to do everything we could to help him. Harry, however, was *full* of cancer," he somberly continued. "Much more than we had anticipated. There were no other tumors found, but there were many small cancerous cells found on his spine, which is not a good place to have them. We couldn't safely remove them all. Since some cells were left, it's likely they'll continue to spread and grow. Also, the tumor that we removed was quite large. Everything took longer than expected, as we were trying to remove as much cancerous tissue as possible. This surgery was quite extensive. Harry handled it all fine, but I can tell you, he is going to be *one hurting cowboy*."

He paused, for a moment, as if to give me a few minutes to absorb what he'd said so far. I just sat and waited for whatever else was coming.

"We do feel, however, because the cells were large in amount but small in size, we can begin treatment as soon as he can tolerate it. He'll be given massive doses of radiation and chemotherapy."

I must have looked startled. I could only imagine what Harry's reaction would be — to that.

Dr. Palmer waited for me to speak. I took a long breath, composed myself and began to ask questions. I wanted to know when they would start the chemotherapy and exactly what those treatments would do. He explained that, in many cases, alternating radiation and chemo treatments helps kill the cancer cells. If all the cancer is eradicated, Harry could have a chance of remission. He did stress, though, that cancer on the spine was a serious place to have radiation. I certainly understood.

I just sat for a moment, overwhelmed with all that had been presented to me. He asked me if I was O.K. and if I would like something to help me sleep. I thanked him, but told him I would be fine. He almost seemed surprised.

"Are you sure?", he again asked. "You've really had a rough day and you're going to need your rest."

I assured him I would be all right and asked when I could see Harry.

"Oh, you may see him now, if you want, but for just a moment. He's in the Intensive Care recovery unit."

We all got up and started down the hall. Suddenly, I frantically turned to the doctor and said, "Dr. Palmer, will you be telling Harry you couldn't get all the cancer— I just couldn't do that."

With a reassuring touch to my arm he nodded. "When Harry is up to it, I will take care of that."

Thank God.

I couldn't imagine how I would *ever* tell him such news.

Gail had been silent all along. She was still holding my hand, which was comforting. As we got up and walked away, she said, "You were so great, Wendy. You were amazing, in such control. I just can't believe how strong you are."

"I'm not so strong, Gail," I sighed. "My knees are still shaking and if you let go of my hand, I'll probably fall down."

I certainly didn't feel strong or amazing, or *anything.*

We walked up to the desk in Intensive Care. I'd never been in an area like that before. All was eerily quiet, except for the soft hissing and beeping of medical machinery. I asked for Harry Kirchner. The nurse led us to a tiny, confined room, just around the corner. It was filled with every kind of stainless steel contraption imaginable. We slowly walked in, with much hesitation. Gail was *still* holding my hand.

I realized why the nurse had come in earlier to talk to us. To prepare *me* — for this.

I stood there, in complete astonishment. Harry lay flat in the middle of the bed, seemingly with more tubes and wires connected to him than a telephone switchboard. He was very pale and seemed *so* small. The respirator tube was down his throat, taking slow, constant breaths for him. I watched the EKG machine monitor his heart. I was speechless.

That picture remains permanent in my mind. Harry lay helpless, defenseless, and so still. It is indescribable to see someone you love in such an incapacitated state.

Gail and I stood in the doorway, leaning on each other. I could bear to watch no longer. "Oh my God, Gail. I can't take this. I've got to go," was all I could say.

"Poor Harry," Gail whispered. We left.

We walked, in silence, to the elevators, rode down to the

main floor, and shuffled through the cold, musty corridor of the parking garage. We were *both* overwhelmed.

Once in front of my car, Gail insisted she wanted to drive me home. She told me George could come back for her car. I stated over and over I was all right. I thanked her several times for waiting with me and hugged her repeatedly.

I drove myself home. Back to our house. Back to my father and to our kids.

Back to a world that would never be the same.

38. . . dying to smoke

Chapter 8

When I walked through the front door, it was nine o'clock. What an unbelievably long day. I raced inside and hugged everyone hello, squeezing them all extra tight. When I asked my father if Harry's mother had called, I was quite surprised when he told me no.

I started for my bedroom as I announced, "Your dad came through the surgery fine. Just let me call your grandmother, as I'm sure she's really worried and waiting to hear from me. Then I'll sit and explain everything to you." I closed the door behind me. I started to shake as I dialed their number. How was I going to tell them this? *More* bad news?

Peggy answered the phone. Before I began to speak, it was apparent that she was upset I hadn't called earlier. I explained I'd just gotten in and told her about the delay. I certainly was sorry she was waiting all day, not knowing what was going on, but I honestly thought she would call my father to find out the details. Nevertheless, I let it go. I knew she was emotionally upset. We all were. But it bothered me deeply that she thought I deliberately didn't call them. I could never have ever done such a thing. *We all* loved Harry. I knew this was difficult for *everyone.*

I began to tell her, word for word, what Dr. Palmer had told me. My voice was soft and quivering.

"Are you saying that Harry still has cancer?", she asked.

"Yes, and the fact that it's on his spine isn't good. It's a very dangerous place to be. They couldn't safely remove it all." Peggy was quiet. I knew this was painful for her to hear. I explained the treatments they were recommending for him.

"When will they start that?", she wondered. I told her they would begin whenever he was strong enough.

Peggy paused for a moment. Her voice was firm, when she next spoke. "Wendy, I don't want Harry's father to know that his son still has cancer. It would be just too much for him to deal with right now."

I was confused. Why would we want to keep that from him? He would be coming down in a week and would certainly find out then. I was too exhausted to dispute it at that time, so I agreed and we hung up.

I sat and thought for a moment. I was *so sad.* Mostly sad, because Harry still had a rough road ahead. Sad, too, that the relationship between Peggy and I was like it was. Instead of helping one another, giving each other support, we were miles apart. Although we had never been particularly close, communication between us had gradually deteriorated over the years. Ever since Harry had been diagnosed, though, things had gotten much worse. I almost felt as though she blamed me, somehow. If only he hadn't married *me*, this never would have happened.

I longed for my mother. I wanted to cry. I wanted someone to hold me and tell me things were going to be all right. There was no one to do that.

If my father saw me fall apart, he wouldn't know what to do. Besides, he was seventy eight years old. In his twilight years, he certainly had a lot to contend with. I know this was painful for him to witness. We'd only moved near him a short four years before. Everything *could* have been so wonderful. Almost from the beginning, though, one thing after the other had gone wrong for us. Wrong for *Harry.*

My thoughts leapt back to the kids. I needed to tell them what was going on. I took a long breath and went to the den. Slowly, in the simplest terms I could find, I explained the situation. I stated that some people do die from this kind of cancer, but the doctors were going to treat Daddy with new kinds of medicines. They were going to try to get rid of the rest of the cancer. I also explained to them, that because the surgery had been so complicated and serious, they wouldn't be able to see their father for a few days, until he was stronger. He needed his rest.

All eyes were watching my every move and expression, so I was careful to smile a lot. I wouldn't be one of those soap opera doctors for *them*. No one had any questions, so I gave everyone hugs and kisses and scooted them off to bed.

Once the kids left, I took my father aside and told him the rest of the situation. He kept assuring me Harry would be all right. There was nothing fake about his comforting. My father really did believe Harry was going to get better. I am certain I receive whatever strength I have from my courageous mother, and my optimistic view from my dear father.

I hugged my father good-night and went in to make some phone calls to friends and relatives who were waiting to hear how Harry was. One by one, I explained the circumstances. We hadn't gone forward with this surgery. We'd taken two steps back.

Harry's recuperation would be long and hard. Radiation and chemotherapy *at the same time*. Harry would need me to be strong.

Above all else, we all needed to have *hope*.

Chapter 9

On Wednesday morning, my father and I went to see Harry. My stomach was in a knot. We walked into the intensive care room and silently watched. There were several IVs, one for blood, one for glucose water, another for the antibiotic. He also had a catheter and the pain button, hooked up and ready for whenever he was. The drainage tube came out of his side, just below his rib cage. It was a big, clear tube, definitely larger than I'd expected. Harry was asleep, but his body seemed restless. His arms were strapped to the rails of the bed. His skin tone was drab, ashen. I watched my father shake his head.

The nurse came in, introduced herself, and gave us a synopsis of Harry's condition. She explained the restraints were necessary, as he'd been trying to pull the tubes out. Most patients try and do that, she said. They're in and out of consciousness and aren't aware of what they're doing. She told us he was doing very well. He'd woken up a few times, but was heavily sedated, as he would be in a great deal of pain. "Harry had a good night," she commented, before she checked his monitors and left.

We stayed for half an hour or so, watching Harry toss and turn. I went over and touched his hand. It lay still, limp. I couldn't believe this was my husband. The man who could do anything, fix anything — go tireless from morning to night, had been reduced to this small, fragile body, lying before me. How could this possibly be happening?

I decided to leave, run some errands and come back later. I dropped my father at home and drove to my bank. I told all my friends at work the not so great news. They were all very reassuring, insisting that Harry would be all right, telling me they've come a long way with chemo. I agreed. I knew in my heart it was true. Despite the odds, Harry was going to be fine.

When the kids came home from school, they were all anxious to hear how their dad was. I told them he was doing better, but was very tired and sleepy. I reiterated they wouldn't be able to visit him for a few days. I wasn't going to let them see him in his current condition. It was frightening enough for me. It would be better if they saw him when at least some of the tubes were gone. I wanted to protect them from as much of the ugliness as I could. Disappointed, but probably relieved, they accepted my decision and took off. How I wished there were someplace *I could run off to.*

Later that afternoon, I went back to the hospital. Harry was awake, but fidgety. The straps, as well as the respirator, had been removed. I assumed that was a good sign. I walked over and gently kissed him on the forehead. He looked up at me and his almost childlike eyes begged me to make this bad thing go away.

"Harry, how are you doing?", I sighed. I took his hand and didn't let it go.

"I'm in so much pain," he began. "I can hardly breathe. Everything hurts so bad. I don't ever remember being in this much pain." How could he? This man hadn't seen the inside of a hospital since he was nine and had broken his leg. He was never even sick with a cold, let alone something like this.

"I know, Harry," was all I could say. "Just try and rest. Each day it will get a little better."

Suddenly, he blurted out a question I wasn't prepared for. In my wildest dreams I didn't think he would have had the strength, or been alert enough, to think of it. "Did they get all the cancer?"

I was stunned. Where was Dr. Palmer? This was supposed to be handled by him, not me! I don't know how my brain thought so fast, especially in my fatigued frame of mind, but somehow I came up with the perfect answer and gave an award winning performance. "They haven't gotten the test results back, Harry. They've sent them to a lab. The doctor will probably have the findings in a day or two," I said convincingly. Wow. I had no idea where that came from, but it sounded so right. It worked. Harry was content and dropped it.

Maybe it was the wrong thing to do. Perhaps I should have told him the truth myself. But my nerves were shot, and I'm sure I would have bumbled a situation that needed to be handled delicately. No, it was the only thing I could have done. The doctor would know the right words, and I would be ready and strong, to help Harry handle the news.

Harry dozed off and on. While awake, his pain seemed unbearable. His face became twisted and tense. It was so difficult to watch. I stayed an hour or so, then quietly left.

I drove back home and had dinner with the kids and my father. They laughed and joked at the table. My mind wandered, no longer participating in the family discussion. Their life was good. Simple. I thought of how great kids have it, but don't know it. Of course, when you're a kid, you don't have life's experiences to point that out to you. So, you just don't know. How I envied them. I wanted to have, my "uncomplicated" life back. No hospitals, no tubes, no cancer.

My mother used to say that life was like a deck of cards. Some people are just dealt a better hand. The trick is, to be smart, play the hand you've gotten, and always look ahead. Well, I decided there were still a lot of cards left in the deck. *I'm in this game, and I won't give up,* I thought to myself. I will not let cancer beat *me*.

That evening, I drove back to the hospital. I was exhausted, but couldn't bear the thought of Harry being there alone. If it weren't for the kids, I'd have just stayed and camped out, but I couldn't do that either. I knew my children needed me just as much as Harry did. They expected me to keep things sane, normal. I felt that was my job. To keep everything *normal.*

Harry was about the same. Sleepy, uncomfortable and irritated. I sat and made small talk for about two hours.

The nurse had brought in a *spirometer*, a small, plastic contraption with tube like channels running up and down. There were numbers on the front and a small red ball inside. Harry was to blow into a strawlike opening on the back and make the ball rise up to the top. This was his homework, she'd said. They wanted him to do this exercise, several times a day, to increase his lung capacity. He wouldn't be allowed to go home until he reached five inches. Harry tried to blow into it, but grimaced in pain. He made the ball reach halfway to one inch and dropped the instrument down in his lap. "I can't do it," he groaned. "I just can't." I knew it was important for him to use this thing, but my motherly instincts wanted them to just leave him alone. Give the poor guy a break. I did encourage him to try, every half hour or so, though without much success.

Harry was exhausted and in a lot of pain. I kept reminding him to push his "pain button" and I was surprised he didn't think to push it much on his own. I don't know if it was a macho thing or if he really didn't remember it was there. I knew he couldn't overdose on it, so a few times I even pushed it for him.

What he really wanted to do was sleep. I left around nine o'clock, talked to the kids for a while, then made more phone calls. I dropped in my bed. As I lay there, listening to myself breathe in and out, I realized how I took that for granted. All day long, deep breaths, short breaths, and they didn't hurt. I stared over at Harry's side of the bed. How I wished he was there, breathing in and out softly, and that it didn't hurt.

My family and friends were a great source of comfort to me during this trying time. There is no question, you really do "find out who your friends are," during a personal crisis. Reassuring support is a necessary aid to people dealing with cancer and the roller coaster your life becomes. We received bags full of food, including whole meals. This was such a significant help, especially since my Dad was "Mr. Mom" and he didn't cook much.

I talked at length, many times, to a girlfriend of mine, Sally, who is a psychiatric nurse. She lived in Maine but we'd kept in touch since we were kids, despite the long distance that separated us. Sally was able to answer a lot of medical questions as well as give me much needed moral support. I guess I am strong, like many people say, but I know that I gathered my strength from the guidance and support of those I love.

Thursday, I went back to work. I didn't want to use up all my sick time and I could visit Harry on my lunch hour, and again at night. How I wished that quitting was an option, but it wasn't. My job provided the entire family's medical coverage and Harry's bills were already piling in.

During lunch, I was surprised to find Harry moved to the "recovery unit". This was a large room, with five or six patients, all with a "privacy screen" surrounding their beds. It was quite noisy in there, considering each patient was hooked up to one or more machines.

I was even further startled to find Harry sitting up in a chair. The nurse was tending to him when I came in. He didn't look very comfortable, almost like a rag doll, somewhat slumped over. He was, however, grinning from ear to ear, quite pleased with himself. This was truly an accomplishment!

"Wow, Harry, look at you!", I cried out.

"Well, it took them half an hour to get me in this chair," he admitted. "But, I'm in it!"

The nurse looked at me and said, rather sweetly, "Yes, well, Harry was quite nervous, so we took it real slow. He did great, though. The doctor wants him moving about."

I sat down and we chatted away. He worked with his spirometer, almost getting it to number two. Another accomplishment.

Harry never moved from his original position in the chair. "I feel like I'm going to break in half," he explained. I went back to work, feeling somewhat relieved. Harry was making progress.

Instead of going home after work, I decided to go to the hospital and have dinner with my husband. It was a good thing I did. Shortly after I arrived, Dr. Palmer walked in. I knew why he was there. Harry was a bit stronger now and Dr. Palmer was ready to drop the bomb. Luckily, I was sitting, as I felt my knees begin to shake. I was holding Harry's hand and continued to do so.

The doctor checked Harry over first and then pulled up a chair. "Harry," he began, "I want to go over the results of your surgery."

I was looking at the doctor, but could see Harry from the corner of my eye. Dr. Palmer was wonderful. He was calm, very direct, but in a gentle way. He told Harry they had found other cancer cells, some on the spine, others in the surrounding areas, but no full spread tumors. He explained the seriousness of those on the spine, but emphasized they were small in number. He then began to discuss treatment. Radiation and chemotherapy. I saw Harry's face drop, but he kept listening. Dr. Palmer explained how radiation was necessary to kill the present cells. The chemo would hopefully prevent future growth. He was very upbeat and reassuring. He did a splendid job.

When he asked Harry if he had any questions, Harry wanted to know when treatment would start.

"When you're strong enough," he answered. There were no more questions. Dr. Palmer shook Harry's hand, told him how great he was doing and left.

Left me to pick up the pieces. What should I say? I didn't have a clue. Then it came to me. I was going to be positive. Encouraging and supportive. Chemotherapy was *not* going to be the end of our world. It was going to help Harry get *well.*

"Chemo," he muttered. "I can't believe I have to have God-damned chemo."

"I know, Harry," I said softly. "But they've made a lot of progress with chemo now. It doesn't make people as sick as it used to. And, if it's going to help you, then that's what you must do." I paused and then said firmly, "You'll be fine Harry, I know you will."

Harry was quiet after that. He had a lot on his mind, and, once again, he chose to handle it in his own way. He wanted to think it all through, alone. I stayed while he ate a little dinner, then headed for home. There was nothing more I could say.

When I arrived home, I walked into what appeared to be the aftermath of World War III. My father had offered to take the kids out to eat. He told the three of them to pick from a McDonald's, Burger King, or such. Apparently each child came up with a different place and a full-blown argument erupted.

This sort of thing made my father crazy, (not to say that it wouldn't upset me also!) He made the final decision, selected Wendy's and told them all to get in the car. Chris' "German" kicked in and he'd refused to go. He had marched himself into his room and closed the door. Of course, this greatly upset my father, probably feeling if he didn't come and eat, Chris would starve to death. An argument through the bedroom door ensued for ten minutes or so, until Chris won the war, stayed home and my father left with the girls, hungry and irritated.

They'd only been back home a short while when I came in. Chris and my father were in Chris' room, again hashing it out. I questioned the problem. Kerin and Kate eagerly offered an explanation, simultaneously, of course.

I was furious. I completely lost my temper. I flew into Chris' room in a fit of rage. He was lying on his bed and, although I startled him, he continued to lay there and continued to defend the fact he did not want Wendy's. I screamed at him for giving his seventy eight year old grandfather a hard time, and for being disrespectful to us both. Of course Chris should have gone with his grandfather, but the situation got blown entirely out of proportion. Everyone's nerves were frayed.

One of Chris' vertical blinds had fallen off the track and lay on the floor. I picked it up, originally with the *normal* thought to hang it back up. In a split second, however, I began to hit him on the leg with it. The blinds were backed with PVC, and since they were quite old and brittle, it shattered. I continued to hit him with it, totally out of control. Sadly, it cut Chris on the leg in several places. Superficial scratches, but blood began to drip before I realized what I had done. My poor father stood there, not knowing what in the world to do. I certainly had taken an unpleasant situation, and made it one hundred times worse.

I realized later on I was not just mad at Chris. Only minutes before, I had left my seriously ill husband, who had just received the second worst news of his life. I was mad at the world, God, and *everyone else* I could blame for this horrid mess.

I ran out of the room, through the house, and took solace behind my door. I wept for thirty minutes. Once I calmed down, I was so ashamed of myself. How could I do such a thing? What was the matter with me? I thought I must be losing my mind. More or less, I guess I was.

Later that evening, I went back to Chris' room. He was sleeping. I sat on his bed for a while, watching him, observing the freshly placed Band-Aids. Tears ran down my cheeks, as I began to speak. I tried to tell him how sorry I was, what stress I was under, how awful I had behaved. I asked for his forgiveness, like I was the child and he, the parent. At some point during my speech, he sat up and hugged me. We stayed that way for a long time. I guess he did forgive me, and I can only hope he understood.

I'd promised myself I wasn't going to let this cancer get to me. It was then I realized, it already had.

Chapter 10

On Friday, during my visit with Harry on my lunch hour, he seemed to be a little stronger, but still in a great amount of pain. His stitches were healing, which meant they were pulling and itching. I took a quick peek at the incision. The slash went from below his rib cage on his right side, across his back, to the tip of his left shoulder. It looked as though they had virtually taken his shoulder off and sewn it back on. Perhaps they had.

It certainly *looked* painful.

He couldn't seem to get comfortable. He grimaced with every move. I tried to help, but it was hard for me to know which position would cause less torment. I encouraged him to eat; he told me he wasn't hungry. I reminded him to use his pain button; he reminded me I was a pain in the ass. Harry was at the end of his rope. He was sick of being in bed and sick of being sick. Unfortunately, I didn't have the power to make things better.

I went back to the hospital, after having dinner at home. Harry's frame of mind was a little better, a little more forgiving of his situation. I asked him if he'd like me to bring the kids the next day. "They really miss their Dad," I told him. He agreed he was now feeling up to seeing them.

"No one else, though," he said, "I don't want anyone else seeing me like this." I guess it was his pride. They had removed so many bits and pieces of him he was no longer feeling whole.

After racing around Saturday morning, doing only the "necessary" cleaning, we all went to see Daddy. I tried to prepare the kids, explaining he was still very weak and full of strange tubes. I, like the nurse, wanted to give them a visual picture, before they walked in and saw him. I also made it very clear there would be *no* jumping onto Daddy or on his bed, and *no* bickering amongst themselves. Be quiet and be *good.*

One by one, the kids slowly entered the room. Harry lay there smiling, a little apprehensive he was about to be pounced on. Each one carefully leaned over, and gave him a kiss hello. There was a moment of awkward silence, which I broke into, talking about some of their latest activities. Curiosity got a hold of Chris, as usual, and he began to inquire about all the tubes and their purpose. The kids all groaned, of course, after hearing about the catheter. After the initial shock wore off, they all began to chatter, almost causing a ruckus. We left Chris alone, while the girls, my father, and I went to the snack bar to get a treat, including a Snickers bar for Daddy.

Once back, we stayed an hour or so, then left for home. It had been a good visit. Harry had put on a good show.

Saturday night, I returned to the hospital. We watched television, occasionally commenting about the show. It was almost like we were home. Almost. Each time I would leave, I would tell him how much I loved him and cautiously give him a hug. I always felt so guilty going home. I hated the fact that I could leave and Harry couldn't.

George had phoned while I was out. I returned his call and updated him on Harry's condition. He wanted to know if he could visit him the next day. I remembered what Harry had said and told him Harry really didn't want any visitors. "Oh, that doesn't apply to *me*," he laughed, "I'll be there in the morning."

George surprised Harry the next morning and of course Harry forgot all about his comment. I'm sure there were lots of off color jokes and plenty of laughter. George would see to that.

After he left, Harry called me. I was busy making beds, tidying up. I was so surprised to hear his voice.

"Is everything all right, Harry?" I questioned.

Harry was ecstatic. "I walked today! The orderly came in while George was here, they both helped me up, and I went up and down the hallway. Twice!"

Hearing the enthusiasm in his voice was a delightful change. "That's wonderful, Harry," I cried. "You must feel great." He then asked when I would be there. Maybe Harry was beginning to feel whole again.

We spent Sunday afternoon and evening, walking up and down the hospital halls. I couldn't help noticing patients in other rooms, some better off, some worse. "I may be able to go home Tuesday," Harry reported happily. I was surprised, but relieved. This part of the nightmare would soon be coming to an end.

I continued to encourage him to use his spirometer. He could now blow the little ball to three, with great difficulty and determination, but it got there.

When I got home Sunday evening, I gave Peggy and Harry Sr. a call. I'd talked to them periodically during the week, keeping them abreast of his recovery. I told them he would probably be coming home on Tuesday. They had packed ahead of time, waiting for my call, so they could leave right away. They were coming to help me take care of Harry.

As we were about to hang up, I remembered Peggy's comment about not telling Harry Sr. of the new cancer. I explained to her that just wouldn't be possible. How could I tell the children not to tell their grandfather Harry still had cancer? They'd certainly think we were trying to hide something. I didn't want to confuse them any more than they were already. I wanted to be completely up front and honest with them. I wanted them to understand that even though their father still had cancer, we all still had hope. Peggy was not happy but agreed. I apologized but I knew I had to do what was best for the kids and for us as a family.

I spent Monday evening with Harry, his last night in that God forsaken hospital. Although he still couldn't move around much, without extreme discomfort, he was definitely more mobile. The only tubes remaining were the drainage tube and an antibiotic IV. Pain pills now replaced the infamous button. He still needed help getting in and out of bed, but once out, he could walk on his own, although he was wobbly and unsteady. Quite an improvement from a week ago. I was amazed, and so very proud.

The nurses left us alone and allowed me to stay past visiting hours. I had taken off from work the next day.

We watched Johnny Carson together as we usually did at home. I remember it vividly because the actor Michael Landon was on. It had been reported that he had liver cancer and he had decided to go on the Tonight Show, to put an end to the nasty rumors that he was dying. Apparently, he chose Johnny's show because they were good friends. Harry and I listened to his comments, hanging on his every word. He did look thin and somewhat haggard, but his spirit was upbeat and confident, just the same. He explained he was trying "holistic medicine", which included healthier eating, massive doses of vitamins, and a spiritual, positive attitude.

Michael Landon had always been a favorite of mine. As I listened, I thought of how strange it was that we all had this unfortunate disease in common. Cancer shows no mercy, no matter how famous you are or how much money you have.

His unquestionable faith in himself was so uplifting. I sat and listened and thought to myself, *if he can do it, Harry, so can you.*

When Michael Landon quietly passed away in his home, on June 1, 1991, the whole country mourned. What a setback for his beloved Hollywood. And for us.

Chapter 11

Exactly eight days after Harry's surgery, I brought him home. As we drove up the driveway, Peggy and Harry, Sr. were sitting in their car, waiting for us. It was obvious they were thrilled to see their son. After many kisses and hugs, we went inside and Harry carefully sat on the couch. He remarked how great it felt to be out of that place and back home. I got everyone cold drinks, while we sat and visited.

After an hour or so, the doorbell rang. It was George. He was off on Tuesdays, so he decided to stop by. He was his old self, joking and entertaining. Although Harry looked tired and uncomfortable, George's stories still made him laugh.

After George left, Harry went in to lie down. I helped his parents get settled in. I had yet to put clean sheets on their bed, as my father had just left that morning. How I had wished he didn't have to go! But Harry's family was there to help now. I knew, in my heart, that was the way it should be.

Later that afternoon, Peggy asked Harry to show her his incision. I still hadn't seen it completely either. He unbuttoned his shirt, and turned around, revealing the huge scar. The staples they'd used to close the wound were still in place. It looked red and sore. Harry's mother looked quickly, then turned away. I know this was painful for her to see. This is not something you expect your son or daughter to ever have to deal with. This truly was a difficult, horrible situation for *everyone*.

The kids came in from school and gave their Dad a grand welcome. One by one, the bookbags opened, showing him their latest accomplishments. We were a family again.

Harry didn't sleep well that night. He was to take his pain medication every four hours, but it wore off sooner than that. He couldn't get comfortable, and tossed and turned all night long. When I got up in the morning, he was already awake, sitting with his parents at the kitchen table, reading the morning paper. I kissed him hello and asked him how he was feeling. "The stitches are killing me and I couldn't sleep," he sighed.

I gave him a hug and told him things would get better. "Just think how far you've come in a week, Harry." I cringed just thinking about it.

Harry began spending a lot of time in bed or lying on the sofa. He appeared very weary, and somewhat depressed. I know he was still hurting badly. Later that night, he again complained about the stitches. I encouraged him to take his pain medication, as it would also help him sleep. I reminded him to use the spirometer that the hospital had sent home with him. He was still struggling to reach "5". This was important, the nurses had told us, as it would help to strengthen and develop the weaker lung. "I hate that thing," he snapped.

"I know, but"... Before I could say another word, he was under the covers and watching TV. I knew he wanted me to leave him alone.

Harry called me at work the following day. He told me the stitches felt swollen and were still painful. I had no idea if this was normal. I told him I'd call the doctor and make an appointment for him to be seen.

The doctor could see him that afternoon. Peggy agreed to take him, so I didn't have to leave work.

When I got home from work, I was anxious to hear how things had gone with the doctor. Harry told me that, although it was still uncomfortable and sore, the doctor felt it was healing normally and was actually doing quite well. They gave him a prescription ointment to help soothe the itch and pain. He seemed to be happier, knowing it was healing so well.

That same evening, Kate reminded me of her upcoming birthday. I had completely forgotten it was on the following Monday, May 20th. She would be eight years old.

"You promised I could have a pool party, Mom. I have to give the kids their invitations," she pleaded.

I stood there, stunned for a moment. I couldn't believe I had forgotten my own daughter's birthday. I dreaded the thought of arranging a party at this late date. "Oh, Kate," I warned her, "I don't know if Daddy is up to having a party here now." I felt so guilty. I'd made it a point, since each of them had been born, to celebrate their birthdays in a big way. I've always felt that, even though everyone loves Christmas, your birthday, well, that's *your* special day. I'd promised myself I would keep things as normal as possible. How could I deny her this party? I went in and talked to Harry.

At first, he was reluctant. "I don't feel like having ten other kids running all over the place," he moaned.

"But it's her birthday. She's turning eight. It's her special day. Besides, I'll keep them out of your hair," I vowed.

Harry smiled and agreed, so I rushed to tell Kate.

We quickly threw together some hand made invitations, for her to give out the next day. Somehow it all got done and ready. Friday night, as I was inflating balloons, Peggy commented that she didn't think we should be having a party right now, especially since it was Harry's first weekend home. Perhaps she was right. Maybe we should have postponed it, or held it at a bowling alley, or a McDonald's. I tried to explain to her my children always had their parties at home and I was desperately trying to keep their lives as normal as possible. I knew Harry didn't want the cancer to change our lives any more than it already had.

The party went on, and all went fine. Harry came out for

the lighting of the candles, had a small piece of cake, then retreated back to our room. Right or wrong, Kate turned eight in a very special way.

The days were busy and went by quickly. I had to work late almost every night, as we were very short-handed in the bank. Dinner was always prepared when I arrived home. Peggy made a comment about not wanting to take over my kitchen, but that I was at work anyway. In the beginning, it was helpful and I did appreciate the assistance.

However, in time, I began to want my kitchen, my family and *my life* back. Things were beginning to get stressful, but as hard as it was, I didn't say a word.

Harry and I began to take long, relaxing walks at night. The evenings were still somewhat cool and it felt wonderful to get out and away. He couldn't walk very fast, but we enjoyed the much needed time alone.

The following week, I managed to get home relatively early one afternoon. Harry was sleeping on the patio lounge chair in our screen room. A heavy afghan lay spread over him. It had to be eighty five degrees. He looked like a little old man. Already pale and drawn, this wasn't helping one bit.

As I took the blanket off, Peggy came out and told me to leave it on. She claimed Harry shouldn't get any sun because he might get skin cancer. *Skin cancer*? That was the least of his worries at this point. I tried to explain that Harry's color was bad. He needed to be outside several times a day. He should also be swimming in the pool, exercising his shoulder; moving around. This would not only be good for him physically, but would lift his spirits as well. How was this laying around doing him one bit of good?

I retreated to my bedroom. A short while later, Harry came in. I told him we needed to talk. I couldn't take it anymore.

I quietly but firmly blurted out all my feelings, one by one. As usual, he listened but said little. Poor Harry, stuck between two strong-willed women, who drastically disagreed on what was in his best interest. He was in an awkward position. He agreed that his mother was treating him like a child and he needed to begin to do things for himself again. We both knew her intentions were good, that she loved her son, and desperately wanted to see him get better.

Unfortunately, our different ideas were slowly pushing the already fragile relationship between Peggy and I further apart. Most importantly, the already stressful situation in our home was getting worse each day.

The following afternoon, Harry had his checkup with Dr. Deligdish. He hadn't seen him since his surgery. I picked him up at home during my lunch hour, since he still was not allowed to drive.

As Dr. Deligdish observed Harry walking in, he commented, "Harry, you're so pale, are you getting outside at all? You need to be out in the sun, take small walks during the day."

I stood and listened. He wanted to know how much activity Harry was getting during the day.

"I rest most of the day," Harry quietly stated.

Dr. Deligdish made it very clear that was to stop. He wanted Harry to keep himself busy, as much as possible. I asked him if swimming and exercising in our pool would be good therapy. "Absolutely," he remarked. "swimming would be wonderful exercise for his shoulder. Water therapy would be extremely helpful."

The doctor told us Harry's incision had healed wonderfully. He would be scheduling chemotherapy and radiation to begin in a week or two. This was not good news for Harry, but I was anxious for it to begin. I wanted it to get rid of those cancer cells fast.

When we got home, Peggy wanted to know what the doctor had to say. Harry told her the doctor wanted him to take several small walks a day, not only for exercise, but to get some sun. He mentioned he was not to lie around any longer, but to keep occupied. Peggy turned and walked away. Perhaps she thought I'd told him to say that. Didn't she understand I wouldn't get any satisfaction in telling her I told you so? I only wanted what was best for Harry, and certainly to listen to the doctor's advice. Whereas we were all in agreement on that, we simply could not seem to communicate it to each other.

I often thought that someone else, facing Harry's situation, more than likely would have a job to go back to by now. Getting out every day, going to work, being productive, is so necessary for one's self esteem.

Later on, during Harry's illness, I met Glen, a young man who had a cancerous brain tumor. He told me his boss had assured him his job would be waiting for him, whenever he felt well enough to come back. He started with a day or two a week and gradually worked his way back to full time. *That*, he firmly told me, had helped his feeling of self-worth.

Sadly, Harry had no job to go to. Truthfully, that made *everything* much worse.

I began to give Harry "chores" to do, while I was at work. Simple things like folding laundry, making lunches, helping get the kids off to school. It didn't compare to a nine to five job, but it helped him feel needed and useful. I also began to go into work a little earlier, so I would be able to finish up and get home earlier to start dinner. I needed to take control of my life again.

Memorial Day weekend, George and Gail invited us to a barbecue. Peggy and Harry Sr. had made plans to visit some friends on the West Coast, so we decided to go.

George met us at the door with a surgical mask on. If anyone else were to do such a thing, it wouldn't have been funny. But Harry roared with laughter too! It was almost like old times. He even had one beer.

On Monday, Memorial Day, Harry's parents were back.

Harry and his father decided to go to Home Depot to buy a screen door. Harry must have mentioned that when he was feeling better, he was going to get one and put it up. He felt it would be so much nicer to be able to open the front door and enjoy a breeze. Apparently Harry's parents offered to buy one for us and his Dad wanted to hang it for him. We both appreciated this very much and told them so.

Later in the day, I was taking a swim with the kids. It felt so good to unwind! I hadn't been in the pool in weeks.

Suddenly, Peggy came bursting through the patio door. "What on earth are you letting him do?" she shouted. I had no idea what she was talking about. Apparently, Harry Sr. had been trying to hang the screen door and had cut it crooked. Harry, the perfectionist, had taken over and was finishing off the bottom with an electric saw. I'd been in the pool for a while, and was not aware of what was going on in the garage, or anywhere else in the world for that matter. Peggy was angry, and told me Harry shouldn't be doing such stressful things.

I looked her right in the eye and told her what I truly believed. "Harry should do whatever he feels like doing. It's important that he see himself as needed, as necessary. He has to keep busy." She glared at me and walked away. From that point on, until they left, Peggy and I spoke very little to each other.

The following week, Harry told his parents that, while we greatly appreciated all their help, the fact was, he was feeling better and could now take care of himself. We both knew they meant well, but it was time for them to leave. We needed to have what was left of our "normal" life back. Twenty six days after they arrived, Peggy and Harry Sr. left.

Dr. Deligdish's office called that afternoon. Harry was to start chemotherapy the following Monday.

62. . . dying to smoke

Chapter 12

Harry's first chemotherapy treatment was on June 10th. During an overnight stay at the hospital, he received *sids platinum*, a fairly common type of chemotherapy used for lung cancer. I stayed with him until they were ready to start administering it, intravenously, about 11 p.m. He was also given a sleeping pill, so he wouldn't be awake while it was going through his veins.

The following day, on my lunch hour, I picked Harry up and asked how it went. His description was quite vivid. When the sids platinum first began to go into his body, it felt like the tip of every extremity was on fire. His fingers, toes, head, even his penis, burned so badly, the pain was excruciating. He said it only lasted two or three minutes, but that's a long time, when you're in that kind of agony.

Harry wore a patch behind his ear, similar to the ones for seasickness, to help prevent nausea. He seemed tired, but all in all, his spirits were good. Once home, he went in to lie down and I went back to work. Over the next few days, Harry was nauseous. He may have vomited once or twice, but nothing too violent. Mostly, he had no desire to eat. His meals were quite small and I would have to remind him to eat or he wouldn't. Remembering my "morning sickness," I was especially sympathetic. I assumed, in time, his appetite would increase. I never expected it to get worse.

The following Sunday was Father's Day. We all went out for breakfast and Harry managed to eat a small amount, probably to be polite. When we arrived home, the kids were anxious to give him their presents. My father had taken them to the local drug store and let them make their own selections. There would not be any shirts and ties for work, this year, but instead, more practical type of gifts were given.

Chris had found a nice, new flashlight and Kate picked a shiny new pen along with a crossword book. Kerin's gift was a profound reminder of how the perception of her father had changed. She'd picked out a small, plastic, three-legged table, usually for outside use. She said she thought it would be nice for Daddy to have next to his bed, so he could put a drink or snack on it, and not have to get up to eat. She volunteered to be his "waitress" and bring his things to him so he could rest. Harry took her up on her offer. That table got great use.

While we were at one of Harry's check-ups, I noticed a small pamphlet hanging on a bulletin board. The cover read, *"Friend to Friend"*. "*A support group for anyone touched by cancer.*" I asked the nurse if I could have one. Surprisingly, it was the only one they had, but she suggested I copy the phone number down. I did and called that day. A pleasant, gentle voice at the other end of the line told me the group met every other Tuesday, in the Radiology wing of the hospital. She encouraged me to come and I told her I would.

Harry, however, didn't want to go. He flatly refused. "I don't want to sit around and talk about cancer," he said. "That's the last thing in the world I want to do."

I tried to convince him several times, but it never worked. He was having a hard enough time sharing his feelings with me, let alone complete strangers. But I found the meetings so supportive and helpful, that I wound up missing just one session during the six months I attended.

Other than Glen, the young man with the brain tumor, I was the only "youthful" person there. The median age was between fifty and sixty. The people I met were extremely warm and caring. One by one, they took me under their wing and made me feel quite welcome. I tried to explain why Harry wouldn't come. They understood and encouraged me to attend anyway. Most of the people there were cancer patients and their spouses, either presently in treatment, or in remission. Those people were especially encouraging and upbeat to listen to. They confirmed the fact that people really do survive this awful disease.

Each night, as we met, we greeted each other with a hug; then another hug good-bye. I made a lot of friends, some of whom I'm still in touch with today. More loving and thoughtful people I have yet to meet.

During the month of June, while I was paying some bills, I came across a certificate that Kate had won. I'd forgotten all about it. She had drawn a "Pizza Hut Playground" in a Pizza Hut coloring contest and won third prize. Four tickets to Miami Seaquarium. She was so proud, as we all were. Nonetheless, these tickets expired the end of June, which was right around the corner. What a shame it would be to not let her take advantage of her winnings.

I approached Harry about it, even though I was sure he wouldn't want to go. He surprised me, however, by saying that he did. I guess he really wanted to get away from it all for a weekend. Chris decided he would rather stay home with his grandfather, so the four of us headed south for some much needed R & R.

We made plans to stay overnight at my cousin's home, in Fort Lauderdale. Our trip to the sea park went well. We took it nice and easy and didn't push ourselves, for Harry's sake. The last morning we were there, I noticed Harry's pillow and the surrounding sheets, were full of loose hair. We'd slept in my cousin's bed, so I quickly took the sheets off, shook them out and put them in her washer. Since Harry had an extremely thick head of hair, on him, it wasn't that noticeable. But sure enough, one chemo treatment and he was losing his hair. The nurses had told him, however, that some people's hair only thins out, then stops. Since he had so much hair, Harry assumed this would probably happen to him and I agreed.

Radiation therapy started the following week. For the next four to six weeks, Harry would be getting the radiation and chemo simultaneously. The only hope of stopping this cancer's growth was to treat it aggressively.

The morning of Harry's first radiation appointment, he called me at work, his voice frantic. "I have to talk to you!", he cried. I hurried into the lunchroom, scared to death to hear any more bad news. "They had me sign a paper, stating they cannot be held responsible if I become paralyzed after radiation. They have to radiate my spine, which is very dangerous." I was shocked, but continued to listen. "I told them that I would refuse to have it then, and do you know what they told me? They said if I don't have the treatments, I have a huge chance of becoming paralyzed. The cancer cells will continue to grow on my spine and form a tumor, which will cause paralysis. Do you believe it? Those are my options! *Maybe* become paralyzed or *most definitely* become paralyzed. Great, huh? I just can't believe this shit."

I didn't know what to say. How much more could this poor man take? Harry, in a wheelchair, was unimaginable — not such a young, active man. "Harry," I cautiously chose my words, "you're right, those are terrible choices, but you know you have to take that risk. The radiation will kill the cancer cells, so that *has* to be done. I'm sure that paper is just for precautionary measures. We have to remain *positive.* It's the only way we can get through this."

Harry was quiet. He agreed and told me they had tattooed "Xs" on his back and chest, marking the spots where the radiation would take place. These tattoos were permanent and were to ensure their aim was precise and accurate. They needed to be permanent, as he would be needing several treatments, over three or four weeks. Poor Harry. After all, even though the tattoos were small, similar in size to that of a mole or freckle, they would always be a permanent reminder of days past.

Think positive, I reminded myself. "You see, Harry," I encouraged him, "they know what they're doing. With those tattoos, they can't mess up." He seemed calmer and we hung up.

I stood there a while, then picked up the phone and dialed Deligdish's office. I wanted to know exactly what was going on, regardless of the news. Amazingly, he got on almost immediately. I apologized for bothering him, which he assured me I was not. I repeated what Harry had told me and wanted his opinion.

Dr. Deligdish explained very cautiously but firmly that Harry's cancer *must* be treated *immediately*. Those cells would, in time, form a tumor which would be both painful and dangerous, with a great possibility of paralysis. I paused for a moment, then suddenly asked him something I knew I had thought about, but had never said aloud. I wanted to know what he thought Harry's chances for recovery and survival were. I desperately wanted to hear there was *still hope*, and although I did not want to hear there wasn't, I *needed to know*. Harry wasn't asking many questions, which I still didn't understand.

The doctor took a moment to answer, perhaps to find the right words. "Harry is an unfortunate young man. His cancer is very serious. This type usually reoccurs within a year, creating the need for more radiation and chemotherapy. If that happens, we would try a new combination of chemotherapy, to reduce or stop the cancer cell growth. Sometimes, the cancer does respond to the treatment, though, and that's what we hope for." *Hope*. There was that word. So there was still hope!

I also wanted to know if Harry's state of denial was normal. Dr. Deligdish told me that fifty percent of his patients want to know everything and fifty percent do not want to know or hear anything that's bad. That is human nature, he said, adding that he tried to respect his patient's wishes. If Harry asked any questions, he would give him honest answers. Until then, he would only tell him what he felt he could handle. I totally agreed. We both had Harry's best interests in mind.

I believe, however, I would be one of the *other fifty percent.* I would want to know, up front, right away. I *think.* Truthfully, though, no one really knows how they would react, until they are dealing with cancer in themselves.

Harry had his second chemo treatment. A few days later, he called me at work, again, completely frenzied. "My hair is falling out — in big clumps. I just took a shower and a whole fistful came out in my hand!"

Within a week, Harry was *completely bald.*

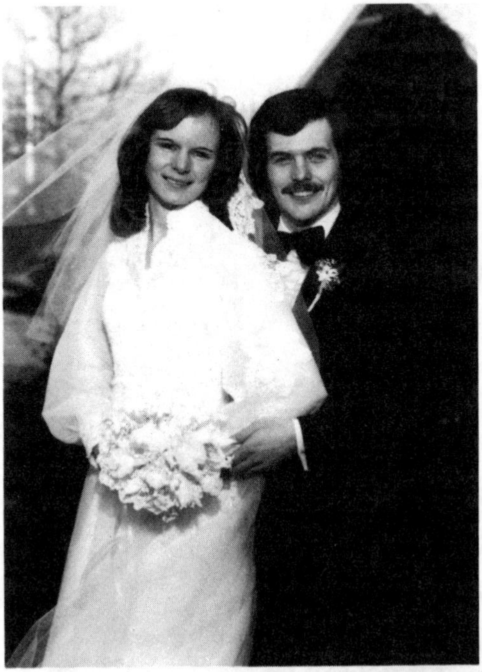

March 20, 1976

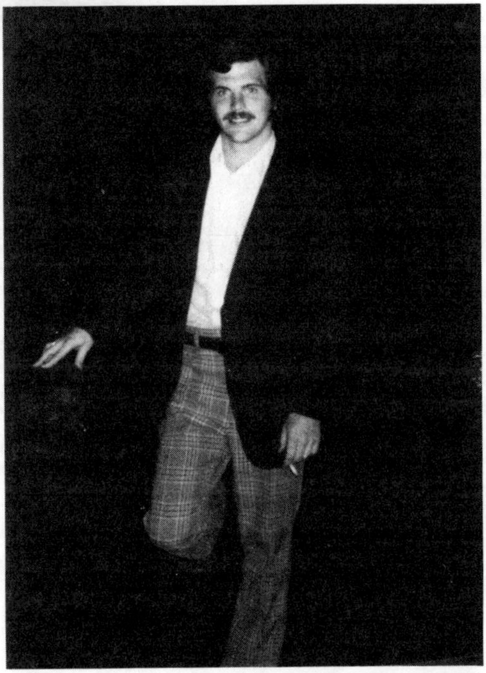

Harry– on our honeymoon in Jamaica.
<u>Note</u>: Cigarette in hand.

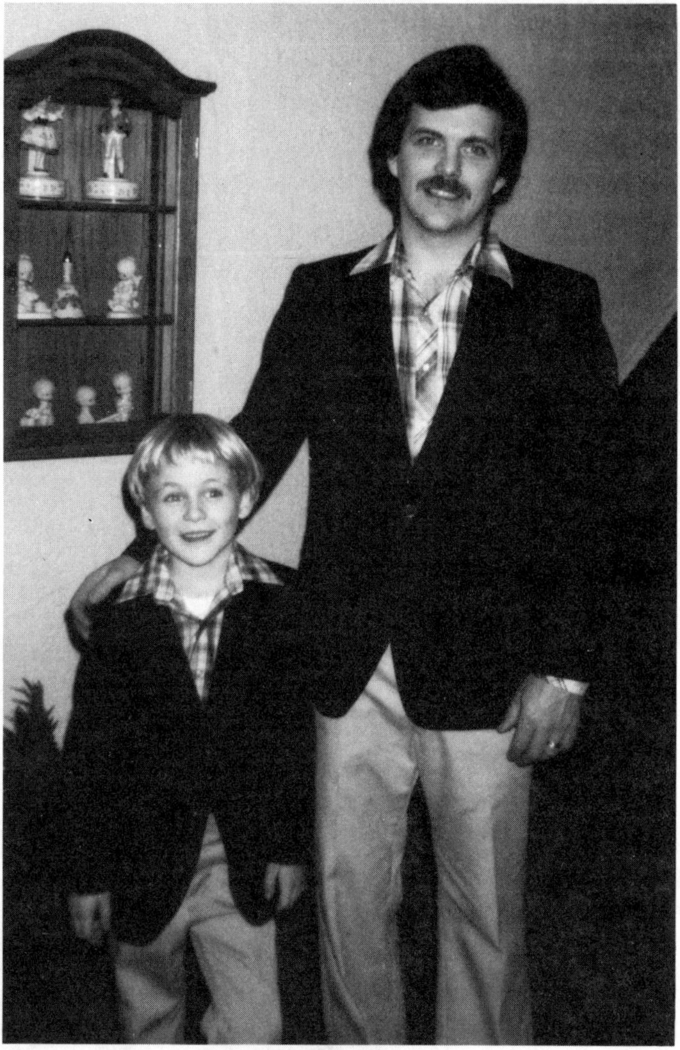

Father and Son,
Thanksgiving, 1983

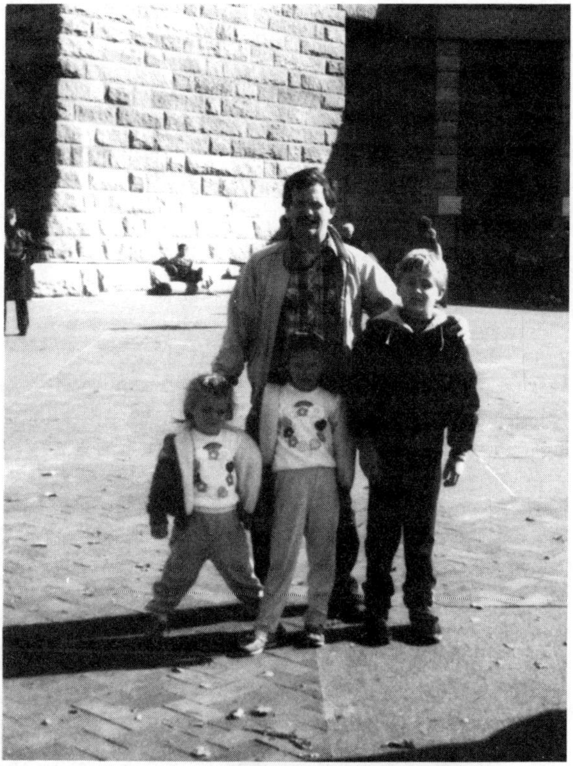

The Empire State Building, March 1987

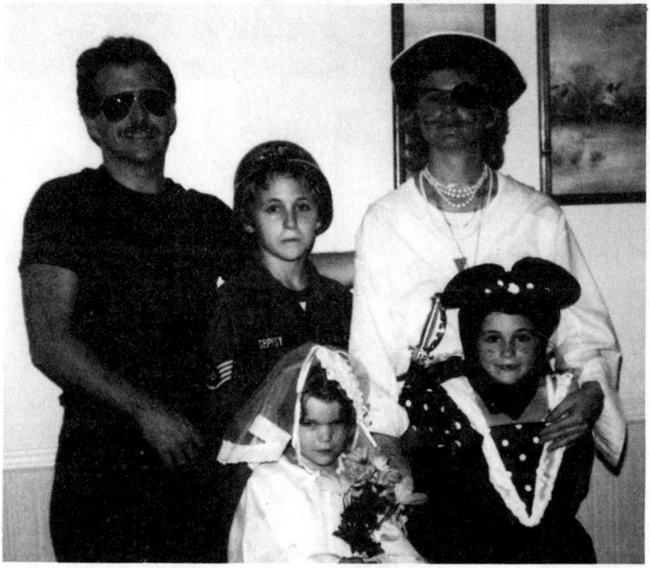

Halloween 1988

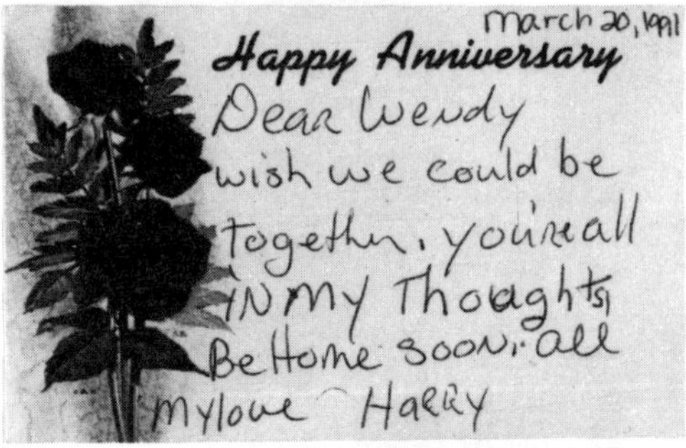

Anniversary flowers, sent from New York.

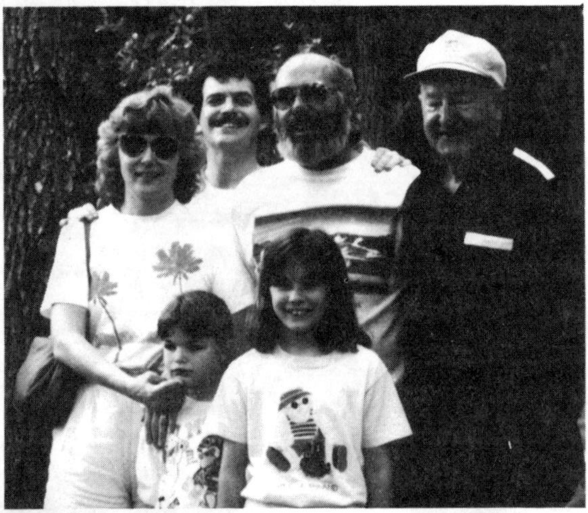

April 1991, Wendy, Harry, Warren, Wendy's Dad Ray, Kate & Kerin. One month before surgery.

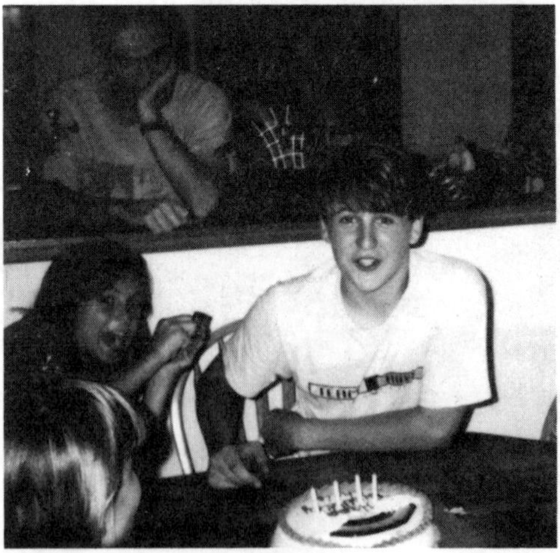

July 1991 Chris' 14th birthday. The beginning of Harry's hair loss.

KIRCHNER, HARRY
FOLLOW UP NOTE
MARCH 6, 1991

DIAGNOSIS: CARCINOMA OF THE LUNG.

INTERVAL NOTE: Mr. Kirchner is seen in follow up today to discuss the results of his needle biopsy which was performed two days ago. I discussed his case with Dr. Smedberg. Pathology revealed a few scattered clusters of malignant cells which were consistent with a carcinoma. Presently, he has no new symptoms. I have recently reviewed the patient's CT scan. A CEA will be performed today.

IMPRESSION: Mr. Kirchner is an unfortunate 37 year old gentleman who presents with a carcinoma involving the apex of his right lung. There are some aspects which suggest that this is a pancoast tumor, although it is not clearly at the apex of the lung. It is a rather large tumor with some involvement of the ribs. It appears to be a squamous cell carcinoma, although there is not a great deal of tissue available for a diagnosis. Given the patient's age, I think he should be treated aggressively and it would not be unreasonable to resect his ribs and chest wall if this were possible for a potential cure. I will discuss this case with a thoracic surgeon. Preoperative radiation therapy certainly needs to be considered at this time. The patient was accompanied by his wife today, and I discussed his prognosis and his options in detail. Given his age and the histology, I have asked for a CT scan of the abdomen and an MRI scan of the brain prior to proceeding with aggressive therapy.

Craig Deligdish, M.D.
CD/pj
Enclosure
cc: Dr. LaRochelle

One of many pages, from Harry's medical file.

74. . . dying to smoke

Chapter 13

In the beginning, Harry was very sensitive about his hair loss. I explained what was happening to the kids, so they would understand how and why Daddy was going bald.

One night, after dinner, however, we were all relaxing around the table. At this point, most of Harry's thick, abundant hair was gone. Suddenly, he looked across at Chris and proclaimed, "I know what I'll buy! *ChiaPet!*" This was a popular child's ceramic item, in which you would plant seeds and grass would eventually grow out of the top. They were usually shaped in different types of animals. Everyone roared with laughter.

For a moment, the old Harry was back, finding humor, even in unpleasant circumstances.

One Saturday afternoon, I came in from grocery shopping, my arms loaded with bags. I looked around for Harry, called out his name, but there was no response. As I entered Kate's room, she and her girlfriend were sitting on the floor, playing a game. When I asked where Daddy was, she told me she thought he was outside. Leaving the groceries on the table, I went out back to search for him.

As I walked into our backyard, I spotted him, hiding behind the children's playhouse. Desperately trying not to be seen, he was crouching, with a cigarette in his mouth. I stood there for a moment, stunned, until his eyes met mine. Every emotion raced through my body. Anger won and my blood ran cold. Without saying a word, I turned and marched back to the house and into Kate's room. I announced firmly that it would be a good idea if they went down to Amy's house to play for a while. "But we want to play *here,*" Kate pleaded. I repeated my statement, a little louder than the first time, Kate got the idea and off they went.

Harry walked into the den, the old familiar cigarette stench still fresh on his clothes. He sat on the couch, glanced over my way, but said nothing. I sat in the chair opposite him and began my sermon, getting angrier and louder as I went on.

"What in the world are you doing?" I never paused for a response. "How could you even look at one of those things? Don't you realize that it was those damn cigarettes that got you in this mess to begin with? What in God's name is the matter with you?! Everyone's trying to help you Harry — the doctors, the nurses, and me!! We all want you to beat this cancer — don't you? Don't you want to *live*? Why don't you just speed things up, get a gun, and blow your brains out? Harry, you're thirty eight years old and you have a wife and three kids who love you. You have everything in the world to live for. Why on earth would you continue to smoke?!!!"

I began to sob, uncontrollably. My head was so filled with emotions, I thought it would burst. Anger, sadness, betrayal. How could he do this to us? *To himself*?

Harry sat on the couch as I ranted on. He behaved much like a child caught with his hand in the cookie jar, but the consequences were so much worse. Ordinarily, he would've never let me carry on like this, without defending his actions, or at the least, his manly honor. This time was different, however. Not only was he too weak and tired, but he had to know I was right. "I only have one, once in a while... I guess I'm..*nervous*..."

"Nervous?," I screamed out. "Hell, I'm nervous too. I'm running around here like a nut trying to take care of everything and everyone, and *you're nervous*? You should be ashamed of yourself, Harry. Honest to God ashamed of yourself."

There was nothing more I could say. The groceries still on the table, I stomped out the door and got in my car. I had no idea where I was going, but I needed to get away. I wanted to run from a life where I was desperately trying to do everything right, but for what? Did he love us even one little bit? Or life itself? I didn't know. I didn't understand.

I drove along the main highway, which peacefully winds back and forth along the beautiful Indian River. It seems strange, that in my irrational state of mind I chose one of my favorite spots. I must have needed its' serenity, the soft ripples, glistening in the mid-day sun. I desperately tried to make sense of Harry still smoking, but couldn't.

I thought back to happier moments — our wedding day — the birth of our babies. How I wished I could have just one of those days again. Tears streamed down my face as reality set back in. How I missed my mother!! No one to talk to, to cry to. There were no happy days anymore, only the pretense of them.

In time, I calmed myself down. There was nothing more I could say or do. I was sure my ranting and raving had woken Harry up. I decided to mention Harry's smoking to Dr. Deligdish who would definitely reinforce my beliefs. Even if Harry wouldn't listen to *me*, I knew he would listen to him. I was convinced and relieved. I drove back home and went about my business, as usual. Dinner needed to be made, laundry needed to be done. My life needed to be returned to.

At Harry's next checkup with Deligdish, I made it a point to be there. As we sat down, I told the doctor Harry was still smoking. Harry glared at me, shocked I had told on him. Dr. Deligdish's expression was perfect. He looked stunned.

Before the doctor could say anything, however, Harry firmly stated, "I only have one or two a day."

Dr. Deligdish looked directly into Harry's eyes. "Harry...You *can not* have one cigarette a day, you *can not* have even one cigarette a year! Your body is a time bomb, just waiting for cancer to return. You must *never, ever* smoke again. If you feel the urge, chew gum, take a long walk. Anything that will help you to not smoke."

Harry said nothing more about it. I felt better. Dr. Deligdish had voiced my concerns quite emphatically. I was sure that was the end of those cigarettes.

About a week later, Kate came into my bathroom, as we all were getting ready for bed. Apparently she had just seen Harry smoking in the backyard. This had upset and confused her. "Why is Daddy still smoking, Mommy? Isn't that what made him get sick?"

I held her in my arms, and shook my head. "I don't know, Kate. *I just don't know.*"

Chapter 14

The days flew by, each one filled with doctor appointments, work, running kids to and from school and sport activities. I dropped into bed each night, both physically and emotionally exhausted. I wondered if I looked as tired as I felt. I was no longer a person, but a robot, controlled only by the needs and wants of others.

One night, Harry happened to mention talking to his mother earlier in the day. He told me she was annoyed with me. I stood there, quite startled. "What did I do?" I couldn't even begin to imagine.

"She's upset that you don't go to my chemo or radiation treatments with me," he answered.

I was stunned, and furious. How could I go with him? I had a job. I *had* to go to work, every day, whether I damn well felt like it or not. My job was supplying our medical benefits. Didn't she understand that? Did she think I could take time off, just like that, continuously, day after day, week after week?

More than angry, I was hurt. How could she possibly think I didn't want to be there with Harry? I would have given anything in the world to have been able to accompany my husband, wherever and whenever he had to go. However, I couldn't do that. I had no choice. I was juggling taking care of Harry, the house, the kids, and, hanging onto my job.

Noticing I was upset, I'm sure Harry deeply regretted saying anything. He told me he'd defended me, let her know he didn't need anyone sitting there, holding his hand. I stood there as he walked away. I allowed my blood to slowly come down from a boil. I was beginning to feel beat up. I was trying so hard — doing all I could possibly do — giving all I could possibly give. Somehow, it would never be enough.

July 8th was my thirty eighth birthday. Harry had gotten a chemo treatment the night before and had only come home late in the morning. He apologized for not having a card or gifts for me. In the past, Harry struggled to buy me birthday and Christmas gifts, never really knowing what to buy. Somehow, though, he always came up with a sentimental card and thoughtful presents. Certainly, considering this year's circumstances, I didn't want, or expect, a thing.

Harry looked peaked and tired. I made him some coffee and toast and he went in to lie down.

Later in the afternoon, I noticed Harry was gone — his car too. Two hours later, he returned, exhausted but smiling, hiding wrapped packages behind his back. I couldn't believe he'd gone out shopping.

He slowly walked over and gave me a soft hug and a tender kiss. "Happy birthday. I felt so guilty not having anything for you to open." As I unwrapped the gifts, tears ran down my cheek. He'd probably felt sick and weak as he walked from store to store. Of course, he shouldn't have done that. But how totally kind and unselfish that he had. Harry was a person of few words, yet he certainly lived up to the phrase "actions sometimes speak louder than words."

A few days later, I received a card from his parents, with a simple "Happy Birthday," signed, "Mom & Dad". Not to a special daughter-in-law, like I had previously received. No one from his family called me. I only mention this because this treatment, especially from his sisters, was not ordinary. In previous years, they'd always call me on my birthday, and other times as well. Now, more than ever, I honestly felt I needed all the love and support I could get. Most importantly — I needed approval.

Perhaps his family didn't fully understand my situation. Somehow, I had become the enemy. But who had started this war and why? We should have been fighting on the same side. Against the cancer. Not each other. We should have been supporting Harry as allies.

I realize now, no matter what I might have done, there would be no winners in that war.

The kids were home from school for the summer. Harry was beginning to spend more and more time in bed. Under some unwritten, unspoken rule, no one bothered Daddy when his door was closed. I got calls at work. A squabble would break out and the kids expected me to solve it, with my magical-mother powers, over the phone. When I asked where their father was, they didn't know, they thought he was sleeping.

The house was usually pretty upside-down, by the time I got home. When Harry was first home, he'd help start dinner. He was no longer able to do that. The sights and smells of food seriously made him sick. Again, memories from my pregnancies made me empathize. As a result, we were eating mostly fast food or simple, quick meals.

Harry didn't feel much like eating anything, so I tried to cater to him. I would call before I left work and ask what he was in the mood for, but I never got much of a response. He was never hungry. I was desperately worried and frustrated about his not eating.

At one of my cancer support group classes, the subject was nutrition. I listened closely to the speaker that night, carefully taking notes. She told us that cancer patients generally lose their appetite, but when undergoing chemo or radiation, (or both, as in Harry's case) the desire to eat is even more diminished.

While everyone knows we should all eat three well-balanced meals, containing all the four basic food groups, this is not always feasible. These patients should eat what they want, when they want to eat it. If they desire an ice-cream sundae for breakfast, that is what they should have. You can throw an egg in it, or better yet, mix *Carnation Instant Breakfast* with it. This, they told us, contains a lot of vitamins and nutrients, disguised as a chocolate/vanilla malt.

The nutritionist also mentioned these people do much better with four or five small, light meals a day, rather than the traditional three larger meals. Their stomachs simply can't take a lot of food at once.

Another interesting suggestion concerned their eating utensils. It seems that receiving chemo tends to leave you with a "metallic" taste in your mouth, probably stemming from the combination of chemicals it consists of. Since the use of a regular stainless steel fork or spoon greatly irritates this sensation, she endorsed the use of plastic ones.

A nutritious drink called "*Ensure*" was another noted recommendation. It comes in all flavors and tastes much like a milk shake. It replenishes many vitamins and fluids lost from lack of eating. Although it is normally given to the elderly, (it quite literally keeps many of them alive), she highly endorsed its use for cancer patients.

I learned a lot that evening. This made so much sense to me. It certainly described Harry to a "T". I went home with my new information, anxious to tell Harry all about it. He still refused to go to my meetings, but always listened intently when I got home.

I began buying simple foods, like applesauce, Jell-O, pudding, lots of soups. I encouraged Harry to eat a little at a time, several times a day, whenever he felt even somewhat hungry. It seemed to work better. He no longer ate his meat and potatoes he was so famous for, but smaller, easier digested items instead. The quantity he would eat at one time would be equivalent to what I remembered our toddlers' meals to be. A spoonful or two, a little more, later on. But at least it was something. Progress had been made.

And, the plastic fork and spoon theory, Harry said, had been the most helpful suggestion yet.

I do, however, vividly remember my first purchase of the *Ensure*. As I entered the grocery aisle, an elderly woman stood before the display, carefully examining each label, perhaps studying over the flavor selection. I watched this eightyish matron, most likely purchasing meals for her ailing, bedridden husband. As I placed two six-packs in my cart, I couldn't help questioning the reality and reason of why I was there.

Chapter 15

At another of my cancer support group meetings, an attorney was the speaker for the evening. He talked about the importance of having a will, setting up an estate, and most crucial, having all things set up jointly. Although Harry and I had all our accounts, and our home, in both names, we didn't have wills. I knew, even without considering his cancer, the fact that we were a family, with three children to provide for, that we should have a will.

I delicately brought up the subject one night and, as I expected, Harry brushed the idea aside. I was determined however, to change his mind. I mentioned it again, a few days later. To my surprise, Harry agreed to meet with a lawyer and I quickly made an appointment with a probate attorney recommended by a friend.

We drove to the meeting, mostly in awkward silence. Once there, the lawyer was friendly but professional, explaining the need for a will, especially concerning the children. He did mention that I'd told him Harry was ill. Harry stared at him, then stated that just because he had cancer, didn't mean he was going to die.

The lawyer softly replied, "Harry, this has nothing to do with cancer. We are *all* going to die someday, of one thing or another, and you have three children to provide for. Who would care for your children, if something happened to both you and

Wendy at the same time? You need to think about that. You should also make certain that all properties are jointly owned. This just makes things less complicated for whoever is the survivor. It gives you peace of mind, as a husband and father."

Harry listened intently, with little more to say. We thanked the man and I assured him we would be back.

On the way home, we began discussing the issue. I reminded him that his car was in his name alone, as well as, a piece of property in upstate New York that he had meant to add my name onto.

Harry began to get angry. "I am *not* going to die, Wendy. You just don't understand. I am going to beat this cancer and I am going to live. I'll add your name to those things, but I have lots of time. I'll add your name to my car in April, at my renewal, or don't you think I'll be alive then?"

I backed off. I felt horrible. I certainly didn't want to give Harry the idea that I thought he would die. I wanted him to have hope. *I wanted him to live.*

When we got home, Harry went in to lie down, closing the door behind him. I never brought up the idea of the will again. It represented death to Harry. It may not have been smart or practical, but that's how it was. Death was not an option.

I've mentioned before how our senses of humor kept us going, our entire marriage. Live, love, laugh. Whenever we would argue, which wasn't very often, one of us would inadvertently make some sort of smart remark and break the tension with laughter. It usually worked.

When he wanted to, Harry could be hilarious. His humor was dry and often unexpected. Once, while Harry was in his bank managers' position, he faxed over a formal letter to my branch. It stated a management decision had been made — the upcoming bank holiday had been canceled and all employees were to report to work that day. It fooled everyone, including my manager and myself. He really had us going all day. We were complaining and fretting about it, until the assistant manager noticed the "Harbor Federal," the name of Harry's bank, in small print at the bottom of the fax! "Your husband!" was all they could say to me.

A few weeks after his lay-off, Harry had come to take me to lunch. He walked into my office carrying a "*Will Work For Food*" sign, scribbled on a piece of a cardboard box. He had everyone in hysterics even though it wasn't *that* funny to me. When it came to Harry and his warped sense of humor, however, even I had to laugh.

As I said, we could usually find humor in most situations, but things had now changed drastically. I was emotionally and physically drained, and Harry was just plain sick and tired of feeling sick. Gilda Radner put it perfectly in her book, "*It's Always Something,*" when she said, "There is nothing funny about cancer." Period. No matter how hard I tried to cheer him up, I couldn't. This was life and death. Harry's life and Harry's death. There was nothing funny about that.

Harry was slowly withdrawing from us. He began to spend more and more time in our room, the door closed. He slept for hours, the covers pulled way up over his head, the room silent and dark. I realize now he was trying to hide from life, not us, but what message did it send to his wife and children?

Thc kids were home all day and yet they rarely ever saw him. They got their own breakfast and lunch, watched TV, played amongst themselves. There was very little interaction with their Dad, if any. I came home for lunch most days, to find the same thing. When I would suggest taking a walk with the kids, or even sitting outside with them by the pool, he would snap at me. "Leave me alone, I'm tired." He was angry so much of the time, that I limited my conversations with him as well. I didn't want to add any more stress to his day or mine. Our children learned to stay away. Daddy was there, but he wasn't there. The door was *closed...*

Here we were, the middle of summer, in Florida, with a beautiful built-in swimming pool right in our backyard. Even though Dr. Deligdish had recommended swimming as good physical therapy, Harry wouldn't use the pool. Only once had he decided to try it, shortly after his surgery. He desperately tried to lift his shoulder to swim, but found himself flopping around awkwardly. He never tried again.

I encouraged him almost daily, for a while, but finally gave up. I guess he didn't want to experience his inability to do something he used to do so well.

Harry's physical appearance had also begun to deteriorate. He probably weighed about one hundred thirty pounds, having lost about thirty five pounds. He tended to leave his left arm hanging, kind of dangling at his side, unless it became absolutely necessary to use it. He'd lost all of his hair, including his eyebrows. Gone was the dark, thick, bushy mustache he was so well known for. The skin on his face was smooth as a baby's behind. "At least I don't have to shave anymore," he sighed.

The most significant change, however, was his *color.* Whereas Harry, of mostly Irish decent, was not a particularly dark-skinned man, in the summer months, after much outside yard work, he could build up quite a healthy looking tan. At this time, he was pale and anemic, with dark circles under his eyes.

Harry hadn't been in my office most of the summer, due to his chemo treatments and all. One afternoon, he decided to stop by, on his way home from a check-up. I could see the shock on everyone's faces. Although Harry never went anywhere without one of his many baseball hats (we had gotten him one in almost every color), it was very apparent he was bald. Later on, I was told that one girl hid herself in the vault, unable to look at him. It was his *color* that was most frightening, she said. (She and her husband did quit smoking at that time, which was at least some small comfort to me). It was becoming more and more obvious to everyone but me; Harry was a very sick man.

Both Chris and Kerin celebrated their birthdays in July.

Chris turned fourteen on the 16th and Kerin turned eleven on the 28th. Both chose to have a small get together of just a few friends for a pool-party/sleep over. By this point, Harry's presence was pretty scarce most of the time. He stayed in bed and only came out when necessary. Most of our children's friends were unaware of his illness. Chris did mention, after his party, a few of the guys had asked him if there was something wrong with his father. His illness had indeed become obvious. Chris told me he simply said his father had cancer.

Kerin's girlfriends, however, being younger, either didn't notice, or were too polite to ask.

I must mention, however, one incident that sticks in my mind. One of Chris' close friends at the time, Joe, knew of Harry's condition. Whenever he was over, Harry told me, Joe would make it a point to search Harry out, and ask him how he was feeling. Harry was deeply touched by his concern and mentioned it to me several times. Certainly proof that teenagers *can* be both thoughtful and considerate.

I tried so very hard during Harry's illness, to be tolerant and understanding, but I was no saint. Many times, not only with Harry, but with the kids as well, my patience would run thin. I wanted desperately to see Harry try to help himself, but he seemed to have given up. It was very frustrating.

I remember vividly one occurrence, that I am truly not proud of. After work one night, I began to throw some sort of dinner together, at the same time cleaning up the day's breakfast and lunch dishes. The house looked like a tornado had hit it, not once, but twice. Harry was in bed, as usual, and the children were scattered.

He came out, amidst my complaining and grumbling, and I began to cry out, in protest of all I had to do. I needed help. Why couldn't he just supervise the kids enough to put their dishes away, pick up their own clothes, I pleaded. Fold some laundry, go to the grocery store for milk. Harry began to fight back. He told me I should work fewer hours. Tell them I just can't stay so late. *Stay late*? I didn't *want* to stay late!

That was it, I had heard enough. I headed for the door. Kerin and Kate, whose presence I had been oblivious to, chased me outside. "Where are you going, Mommy? We want to come. Where are you going?", they wailed. I gave them a quick, unresponsive hug and jumped into my car, heading for the Interstate, so that I could drive fast. I wanted to run away and never come back. I didn't know how much more I could take of this.

I drove to Vero Beach, where my father lived, fifty miles away. Like a little girl, running home to Daddy, I desperately wanted him to hold me and tell me everything was going to be all right.

As I pulled up, I was surprised to see Chris come outside. My days had been so hectic I'd completely forgotten my father had picked him up a few days before, so they could spend some time together. I began to sob, detailing my woes, from beginning to end.

Chris stood and listened, sympathetically. They both gave me a big hug and we all went inside.

I called home and told Harry I was staying overnight at Dad's and I'd be home in the morning. I apologized and tried to explain I simply needed some time away. His tone was aloof, but surprisingly understanding. He asked me to speak to the girls, claiming they were still upset. They both got on the phone and asked if I was *ever* coming home. How awful for them, that they could even think I would do such a thing! I assured them over and over I was coming back, that Mommy just needed some rest. I asked them what their father was doing and they said he'd gone back to bed. They seemed fine, when we hung up. I spent the rest of the night playing cards with my father and Chris.

Early in the morning, I drove home, showered, dressed for work and left. Harry never mentioned the incident again.

I, however, didn't forget it. I'd run away from Harry, the house, the mess, the *cancer. I* was able to do that. But what about Harry? He had to face the cancer every day, with *nowhere* for him to go. I was determined to do whatever it would take to help Harry get through this and get well. How did I dare make his life more miserable?

I really and truly only wanted Harry to get better. For things to be like they used to be.

I wanted Harry to *live.*

Chapter 16

In August, one of my closest, long-time friends, Claudia, came for a visit, with her twelve year old daughter, Renee. We'd planned a family vacation and decided to include Claudia and Renee as well. Claudia had actually known Harry before I did, since her husband, Bob, and Harry had been childhood friends. Claudia and I met when Harry and I began to date and had been the best of friends ever since.

I'd prepared them as to what to expect. Even though I'd been in constant contact with Claudia, needing her much comforting shoulder to cry on, I still felt that actually seeing him for the first time would be difficult. I expected it to be especially hard for Renee, who had known Harry all her life. At such a young age, it would be quite a shock to see him as he now looked.

Surprisingly, they both did a terrific job of hiding any emotions, other than pure joy to be with all of us.

Harry joked about his hair, or lack of it, whipping off his hat the minute they walked in. That helped to break the ice. I was happy to see Harry so comfortable. Since his illness, we'd done very little socializing, and it felt wonderful to have friends in the house again.

On August 14th, Harry had his last chemo treatment. We all took him to the hospital, stayed a while, then went out to dinner. After I picked up Harry the next morning, he strutted about the house, proclaiming over and over, "No more chemo!" I asked him if he wanted me to go buy a cake, in honor of the "memorable day". Unfortunately, he didn't want one. As happy as he was, it was all over, he still didn't feel much like eating.

Emptying his overnight bag, he handed me his pajamas and boldly told me to throw them away. "I don't want to ever see those again," he said. "I'm finished with hospitals and chemotherapy." I told him I'd give them to my father, but I never did. Although I was also hoping and praying all the treatments were over, I was still very leery and quite concerned.

We had agreed on a trip to the Florida Keys. One of our favorite family vacations together had been to Key Largo, just the summer before. Subconsciously, we must have wanted a repeat of the relaxing, carefree getaway, we had experienced a brief twelve months before. Harry looked forward to the trip as well, mentioning it frequently.

Unexpectedly, the day before we were to leave, Harry changed his mind and told me he wanted to stay home, alone. He insisted we still go, but said he just couldn't see himself sitting in the car for that long and, especially, eating out. I can only assume he thought by that time, he would be feeling better. Unfortunately, he wasn't. He was still tired and uninterested in eating. "I'd wind up staying back at the hotel most of the time, anyway," he told me.

I was quite upset. I firmly told him, over and over, that we wouldn't go without him. But he insisted on it so strongly, I began to realize he really *wanted* us to go. He must have been looking forward to the peace and quiet and, to being alone for a while. Claudia and I talked about it, and decided to go. I felt terrible Harry was not coming, but knew I could really use the break. Certainly, we could *all* use some time apart.

On Tuesday morning, Claudia and I, and the four kids, packed up the car and headed south. We were only gone for four days, but we still managed to get in lots of much needed relaxation and tranquillity. I felt as though I had been temporarily liberated from the difficult situation we were all facing. I felt guilty, feeling that way, so I called Harry twice a day, to try and compensate. He sounded fine and jokingly asked us to stay longer.

Claudia, however, took me aside one day, to voice her concerns. She said she'd seen Harry smoking one afternoon, behind the house. She was both shocked and sickened. How could he continue to smoke the very cigarettes that caused his cancer, at the same time, receive chemotherapy, to help cure it? We cried as we tried to rationalize his apparent slow, suicide. We concluded that Harry did want to live, but in his weakened condition, was so chemically addicted, quitting was beyond his control. What could we do? Dr. Deligdish's words echoed in my head.

Claudia also said she had assumed, since his surgery had been three months before and his radiation and chemo treatments finished, that Harry would be doing better. She felt he shouldn't be so weak and tired. Her biggest concern, however, was the amount of time he spent in bed.

I listened intently. As she pointed these things out to me, I thought about a friend, Pat, whom I had met in my cancer support group. Pat had been diagnosed with uterine cancer and had been receiving her chemo treatments around the same time as Harry. She seemed to have so much more energy and spunk. She was back to work part-time, had gained back some weight, and told me how food was beginning to taste good to her again. Was Harry just depressed because he didn't have a job to go to? Or was he truly as sick and as weary as he appeared?

I mentioned Pat to Claudia. She suggested I call the doctor when we got back. I asked Claudia how many hours a day she thought Harry spent in bed. I thought maybe sixteen. "Wendy, he's in there a lot more than that," she answered. I guess the things that had become so "normal" to me, were far from it. Claudia was right. I had to take charge, stop accepting things as they were. I *had to help* Harry.

The day Claudia and Renee left, I called Dr. Deligdish's office on my lunch hour. He returned my call a short time later. I voiced my concerns and he seemed surprised. "I don't get that impression from Harry at all, when he's here. I've asked him how much time he spends in bed and he told me very little. He also told me he was eating better. You're painting a very different picture. Harry needs to be as active as possible. Laying around in bed isn't good for him, physically or mentally. It will only add to his depressed state of mind. We need to work on this. I'm very glad you called."

He assured me he would talk to Harry during their next visit. I thanked him, once again, for taking the time out of his busy day to talk to me. It was then Dr. Deligdish set me straight. "Wendy," (I liked the fact he no longer referred to me as Mrs. Kirchner), "you are by no means bothering me. How else would I know what is going on? Harry is not leveling with me. Please feel free to call me anytime. We need to be in contact with each other, to be able to help Harry better."

It was at that moment I understood why this doctor, who had in the beginning, seemed distant and unapproachable, won the "doctor with the biggest heart" award. This was the start of many phone calls, which would help me deal with this troubled situation, help me face the difficult challenges that had now become part of our daily lives.

It was reassuring, in this war against Harry's cancer, that Dr. Deligdish and I were fighting the battle together.

Chapter 17

One Saturday evening, I talked Harry into getting out and seeing a movie. It had been months since we'd been out alone. Harry even agreed to eat out first. We decided to use the gift certificate, from Kathy at work. She had given it to us when Harry was in the hospital.

We ate dinner at a lovely, scenic restaurant that overlooked the peaceful Indian River, watching dolphins leap in and out of the water. Together we laughed as a man almost fell in Harry's lap, trying to see the fish as well. Even though he didn't eat much, it was one of the most pleasant dinners Harry and I had experienced in a long, long time.

Foolishly, I had chosen the movie, "*The Doctor*." Although Harry had initially protested that he'd seen enough of doctors, he agreed to see it after I read him the favorable review.

As the story progressed, I realized what an awful mistake I had made! Not only did the doctor, William Hurt, come down with cancer, a girl he befriends at a support group subsequently dies of cancer of the brain. What in the world had I been thinking? I had no idea the subject matter would hit so close to home. I didn't dare look at Harry the entire two hours. Luckily, the ending was a happy one. The doctor's cancer was in remission and he and his wife patched up a troubled relationship. Unfortunately, I didn't choose a very entertaining way for Harry to spend his long awaited evening out.

Late in August, George began to call Harry on his day off and ask him to join him fishing. George knew Harry was alone, now that the kids were back to school, and he was housebound most of the week. The highlight of Harry's outings had now become his doctor visits. George felt it was imperative that Harry get out and refused to take no for an answer.

During these get togethers, no mention of Harry's illness ever took place. Nevertheless, they had to be both beneficial and therapeutic for Harry. He needed diversion and a good friend. George provided both.

The last week of September, my brother, Wayne, came in for a visit from San Diego, California. He had mentioned wanting to visit us all, especially Harry, several times and was finally able to get away from his busy real estate business. I didn't know it then, but he was quite worried about Harry. A friend of his was a nurse and had told him how serious this condition was.

Fortunately, Harry's hair had started to grow back. He still looked tired and frail, but somehow, having eyebrows and hair on his head made a world of difference. My brother probably saw Harry the best he had looked in a long time.

We planned a night out together, including my father, and went to the movie, "*The Fischer King,*" with Robin Williams, one of Harry's favorite actors. Once again, it was not a great choice. The overall mood of the storyline was both bizarre and depressing. One doesn't need to see gloom and doom, when you're cooped up in the house all week. Nevertheless, despite the somber movie, we all had an enjoyable evening out. Almost like old times.

It was wonderful to see my brother and I know he was glad he came.

During the last few weeks of September and into October, I noticed Harry seemed chilly most of the time. It was still quite warm in Florida; we were all in tank tops and shorts, but Harry walked around the house in long-sleeves and sweatpants. He watched TV with an afghan pulled way up to his neck. One evening, he looked unusually flushed and was sweating beneath the blanket. When I questioned why he didn't take the blanket off, he said he was cold. I kept lowering the air conditioning. We were sweltering and Harry insisted he was still cold. When I took his temperature, it was 100 degrees.

Night after night, Harry's condition remained the same. Once again, I got on the phone to Deligdish. He seemed quite concerned.

"Harry should be doing better than he is right now. He shouldn't be running even a low grade fever. I suspect he might have cancer in the bone marrow. I'll order a *bone scan.*" He explained this is a test where a long needle is inserted into the spine, retrieving a sample of marrow, to biopsy for cancer cells.

The doctor felt it was in Harry's best interest not mention this test to him ahead of time. While it can be somewhat painful, there was no point in Harry being anxious about it. I understood, and agreed not to mention it. How difficult that was for me, though!

On the day of his next office appointment, Harry seemed relaxed and calm. I went off to work, knowing full well what was to take place. I didn't like keeping things from Harry, but I knew it was for the best. Nevertheless, I felt awful.

Later that afternoon, Harry called me at work, from home. He proceeded to tell me all about the test, how it was the most painful thing he could remember. He was extremely embarrassed, because he had screamed out in agony. I assured him he had nothing to be ashamed of. After all, if it hurts, it hurts.

I never did have the heart to tell him I had known about it before.

The results of the bone marrow scan were negative. Harry was elated. I celebrated by cooking him a special dinner that night, a steak on the barbecue, which had previously been one of his all time favorites. He surprised me by even eating a little bit of it.

In a subsequent phone call to Dr. Deligdish, however, he informed me he didn't think the biopsy they had taken had been adequate. That could produce a negative result, even if cancer cells were present. "Harry has all the symptoms," he warned me. "The night sweats, the low grade fevers, his high white blood cell count." Harry's recent visits had revealed white blood cell counts of 30,000, 35,000 and most recently 40,000. Normal counts range from 4,000 to 10,000.

Dr. Deligdish advised me to let things be. There was no point in putting Harry through another painful test. By letting Harry believe it was negative, his spirits would be better, which would be a great help in improving his condition. The doctor also added, they would treat him with more chemotherapy if it became necessary. His major concern, however, was getting Harry's white blood cell count down.

The doctor also mentioned he was going to order another MRI. It had been six weeks or so, since Harry's last chemotherapy treatment. It was time to check him from head to toe, to see if any new tumors had formed. "If none are found," he explained, "it will be a good indication the chemo has either stopped, or certainly slowed down, the growth of the cancer."

Once again, things were not great, but there was still *hope*.

A few days after Harry's scheduled MRI, I came home from work to find Harry lying in bed. He didn't rise, as he usually would. I could tell something *was very wrong*. He was completely expressionless. "What's the matter, Harry?", I cautiously asked.

He slowly responded. His voice barely above a whisper. "The doctor called a little while ago... They found a huge tumor on one of my kidneys — so large, it's the size of a grapefruit."

I was stunned, horrified, terrified. In one split second, millions of thoughts ran through my head. After months and months of hoping and praying, telling myself over and over that he would beat this, he would get better, suddenly, all hope was gone. There was no denying it now. Aggressive radiation and chemotherapy treatment, and still, a huge mass had been able to form. I was no oncologist, but, I didn't need Dr. Deligdish to spell this out to me.

My dear God, Harry is dying.

However, in a performance that could seize any academy award nomination, I held my husband in my arms, looked right at his face and told him, "Don't worry Harry...*you're going to be all right*."

Chapter 18

Time had a whole new meaning now. I knew each day was a gift to be well spent with Harry. As much as I wanted to believe Harry would live through this, that we would grow old together, watch our grandchildren play, I couldn't pretend any more. I decided we would be better off living each day to its fullest. If a wonderful miracle should occur, and Harry got better, then nothing had been lost. We would just have many more wonderful memories together.

I knew I had to tell the children. How could I do that, when Harry, himself, was not facing the truth? I didn't know exactly what to say, but I wanted the kids to understand what was happening.

I talked to Chris first. I told him all about the new tumor that had formed. Right away, he knew that wasn't a good sign. "That's bad news, isn't it, Mom?" he asked. I told him it was, but the doctor was going to do whatever he could. Perhaps a different type of chemo would help. I emphasized, however, that the doctor and I *were very worried.*

Chris wanted to know if Dad's tumors were growing because he was still smoking. I was speechless. Apparently, all three children had seen Harry smoking, at one time or another. He hid his smoking from me, but not from them. I shook my head and shrugged my shoulders. I told Chris I had no answers. I think he understood. He had no choice.

The girls and I went out to dinner one night. I tried to slip into their conversation, calmly and gradually. I told them Daddy had a new tumor growing and the doctor and I were concerned about it. The treatments he had been receiving up until now had not been working. Kerin wanted to know if he was going to have another operation. I said I didn't think so, but they might give him a new kind of chemotherapy which might help. I pointed out that we all needed to be extra good and helpful to Daddy these days. I tried to explain that he was very sick and really needed our love and support more than ever. I didn't use the word *die.* I had planned to, but I couldn't bring myself to say that aloud yet. Not to them, nor myself.

The girls seemed to understand, but truthfully, I really didn't know what thoughts were going through their young innocent minds.

My family was living out a nightmare. The saddest of movies. One that usually would bring me to tears, even though I would know it wasn't real. Well, this was real. I was overwhelmed with every emotion possible, totally consumed with the fact that I knew Harry was going to die, but I couldn't talk about it, especially to him.

I would be without him before too long. I would lose my husband, my children would lose their father. Most unfair of all, Harry was going to lose his life. At only thirty eight years old. Why? Why was this happening? We had only begun to live.

I cannot write a book concerning death and dying and not mention religion. Going to God in a time of need can be both mentally and, many times, physically healing. The power of prayer is certainly a strong one. Faith can move mountains, as they say.

Unfortunately, Harry had never been a very religious man. He had been raised Catholic and attended Catholic school during his elementary years, but seemed to have some sort of falling out with his church somewhere along the way. When we were dating, he attended my Methodist church with me many times, and a few more once we were married, but then he stopped. He absolutely refused to go. I went alone for a while, then stopped also, until the kids were old enough to attend Sunday School. From that point on, I went to church every week by myself, after I took the children to their Sunday School classes. Easter and Christmas, Harry would come along, but that was it.

We talked about God, many times. His religious beliefs were pretty common, I guess. He did believe in God, although the whole "religious concept" was just not an important aspect of his life. He was too busy, he would say. I honestly feel that if people have *no* God in their lives, who or what do they answer to? That leaves too much room for unscrupulous, immoral behavior.

Nevertheless, I do believe Harry resolved his conflicts, toward the end of his illness.

Apparently his mother had brought him his childhood Bible, when they came down after his surgery. He had put it aside for a long while, but it resurfaced and appeared on his night stand. I never saw him read it, or even pick it up, but it remained there throughout the rest of his struggle to get well. Since it was so readily available, right next to where he lay, so much of the time, I can only hope, for his sake, he did read it, and gain some comfort from it. I know in my heart Harry needed God's help to get through each day.

There is no doubt, things would have been much easier for us both, if Harry had not been in denial. We could have talked of many wonderful memories together. Although I know we would have shed a ton of tears, we could have cried together, in each other's arms. Instead, I often cried alone, in the bathroom while I showered, so the splashing water would drown my sobs.

Only once, do I remember Harry crying for no apparent reason. It was a Saturday morning, sometime in August, and I was up and about, doing my typical Saturday chores. Harry was still in bed, yet it was almost 10:30. When I went over to ask him if he was all right, I realized he was crying.

I sat on the bed and quietly asked him what was the matter. He slowly, for one brief moment, *let me in*. He told me he was crying because every day was the same. He had nothing to look forward to, except the guarantee that he was going to get up, with nowhere to go, and still feel miserable. I couldn't believe what he said. How awful for him, that this is what life for him had become. I moved closer and hugged him. I told him I was so sorry that he felt this way, both physically and mentally, but I begged him to not give up hope. There was still the possibility the medicine could work. Maybe life was going to give Harry a second chance. At that point, he got up and left, however. That was it for sharing such deep, personal thoughts and feelings. I honestly think he was annoyed at himself, both for feeling those feelings, as well as sharing them. My poor, private Harry. Why should things have been like this? I have no answers.

Harry didn't share his thoughts or feelings with any of his three children either. How proud he was of them, how much he loved them. I can only assume it was too painful for him to face the truth. He was the kind of man who didn't want his children to see him weak or crying. He was *the father*. That would not be under the normal realm of things. However, nothing was "*normal*" anymore.

It is still quite sad for me to admit we never once discussed the fact he might die. We only talked about new treatments, tomorrow, and next week. Claudia believes Harry knew all along he might die, but was trying to protect us.

Perhaps she is right.

Dr. Deligdish wanted a biopsy of the newly discovered tumor. Although he was ninety nine percent certain it was of cancerous element, he wanted a positive diagnosis of the type. This would help him decide what new type of chemo to use. A few days before the scheduled test, I called the doctor. I wanted to know, truthfully, if this new treatment had a chance of working. Perhaps I wanted to hear this new miraculous type of chemotherapy could save my Harry's life.

Dr. Deligdish told me that although there was a chance the tumor would respond to the new treatment, he was baffled by Harry's cancer. It apparently was a very aggressive, fast growing kind. He mentioned he had brought Harry's case before the "tumor board", a group of specialized physicians, who meet weekly and discuss particular patients who have unusual symptoms or circumstances. Every professional opinion is helpful, certainly under life and death situations. Nevertheless, Dr. Deligdish said he was trying to remain *hopeful*.

I was determined to try and do the same.

I took the day off from work to be with Harry during his biopsy test. It was an out patient procedure, so he most likely would be discharged later that afternoon. We waited in his room for quite a while, idly chatting, mostly watching TV. When the nurse finally came for him, she told me the procedure would take several hours, so I probably should go home and come back later. I agreed to go, as I knew I was better off occupying my time and my mind, at home.

Amidst sorting mountains of laundry, the phone rang. It was Peggy, whom I hadn't spoken to in months. Harry had told her of his recent tumor, and the day's test. She asked about the biopsy results. I explained to her, since they were only doing the procedure that morning, we probably wouldn't have the results back for at least a few days. She wanted to know why this biopsy was necessary at all. I tried to explain the doctor needed to know what kind of cancer it was, to decide on the next method of treatment.

Her next question was a tough one. What did the doctor think of Harry's overall condition? It didn't matter that our relationship was strained and uncomfortable — I dreaded answering *that.* Harry was her son, whom she, without a doubt, loved unconditionally. I wanted to answer as compassionately and kindly as possible.

"Dr. Deligdish is very concerned," I cautiously told her. "It's not a good sign that a new tumor grew after all the radiation and chemo treatments he's had."

I guess she read between the lines. The only thing she said, however, was, "Well, *I* still have hope."

After we hung up, I sat there for a moment. All alone, in a very quiet house. Did I not still have hope? Yes, I did. But it was a different kind of hope now. I didn't have much hope for the new cancer-killing chemotherapy. I hoped for a *miracle.*

And miracles do happen.

A short time later, Harry's sister, Joan, called me. I hadn't spoken to her in many weeks. I'd always liked Joan. She was friendly and down to earth and I was happy she called. It felt good to talk to *anyone* who would listen, right then. Joan wanted to know, point blank, what was going on. I knew I had to be honest. I explained the grim details. She listened intently. Finally, in a burst of tears, I told her it appeared Harry was dying. It was the first time I had actually said those words out loud. We both cried and tried to console one another, before we hung up. But there truly are no words, at such a time, that can take that kind of pain away.

I felt horrible telling her such news over the phone, but I had no choice. This was their son and brother. Harry's family had to know.

The hospital called. The biopsy procedure had been canceled. The tumor was apparently too close to vital organs, so it couldn't be done safely. I drove back to the hospital. Harry seemed relieved, yet discouraged.

His white blood cell count was now 50,000. He was still running low grade fevers, hardly eating, rarely sleeping. Several times a night, he would get up, walk around, then get back into bed. He couldn't seem to get comfortable. He continued to sweat profusely, and had begun to sleep on towels. Several times a night, he would get up to replace them with fresh, dry ones. I also put towels on the den couch, because when he napped, he would again wake up drenched.

Dr. Deligdish had decided on the new type of chemotherapy, but he wanted to wait until Harry's white cell count improved.

It was during this time, Harry began talking about going to New York. He commented that none of his brothers or sisters had come to visit him. I was tremendously upset by that, mostly sad for Harry. Five brothers and sisters, how could not one of them come to see their brother? I later concluded they either didn't realize how serious his condition was, or they all simply couldn't face the fact that he might die. Regardless, I wish someone would have come. As painful as it might have been for them, Harry needed all the love and support he could get.

Harry mentioned he might fly up after the holidays. After quick thinking, I told him I was surprised he would want to go during the extreme cold weather, especially since he was already chilly in Florida. He thought about it and agreed. "I guess I'll go soon then," he said. Despite their odd way of showing it, I knew Harry's family loved him and deserved to see their brother and son.

Most importantly, I knew Harry wanted to go.

The following week, I went to the local travel agency and booked Harry a flight. The girls went with me, but played out front, searching through the colorful brochures. As the agent handed me the tickets, I began to cry. Within moments, I blurted out that my husband was dying and I was sending him to New York to visit his parents, brothers and sisters for the last time. I told her I had no idea how I was going to tell our children their father was going to die. I don't know where all the emotion came from. I guess I unloaded days and days of unspoken sadness and grief to a complete stranger. The poor woman. She just took my hand and told me how sorry she was. She was sorry, I was sorry. I was wallowing in pity for us all.

I arranged for Harry to go to New York on Oct. 31st and return Nov.10th. Ten days would do him good, getting away and being with his family. Although I really didn't want him to go, I knew he would be fussed over and well taken care of.

The night before his departure, our local park had a "haunted hayride." It sounded like fun and even Harry agreed it would be a great family outing, before he went away. We got there fairly early in the evening, but the line was already several city blocks long. We waited and waited and Harry grumbled, as usual. He never had the patience for waiting in long lines. A day at Disney was his worst nightmare!

While in line, we ran into Dr. Deligdish's nurse, Jill. She was bubbly and so happy to see us. She knew all about Harry's visit to New York and wished him a wonderful trip.

Towards the end of our wait, Harry looked sternly at me and said "This is the *last time* I'm coming here. This line is ridiculous — next year, I'm staying home." I looked right at him, but didn't say a word. Since then, I've asked myself hundreds of times, did Harry *really believe* he had a next year? I was his wife. I knew him better than anyone. And yet, I truly don't know.

That evening, after everyone had gone to bed, I sat up until 1:30 in the morning, with pen and paper. I wrote Harry a letter. He would be leaving the next afternoon, for ten days, and there was so much I wanted to say. There never seemed to be the right time or place, so I wrote down all my thoughts and concerns, shedding more tears than ink.

I remained optimistic, telling him my one and only wish was that he get well and we all be a family again. I also begged him to *talk* to me, to tell me how he felt about things, to *please let me in.* I just honest-to-God wanted to let him know, no matter what, I was there.

That letter, if nothing else, gave me much needed relief. I had said what I needed to say. I tucked the envelope deep in his suitcase, knowing at some point, in New York, he would come across it and hear my words.

The following day, Halloween, I drove Harry to the airport, dressed in my vampire costume (my branch dresses in costume every year.) He laughed at the sight of me, amazed I would actually drive looking like that. When we arrived, the vampire kissed her husband good-bye and hugged him tightly, for a long time.

As I drove back to work, I thought to myself, *I can't wait for Harry to get back...* I hated for us all to be without him.

Chapter 19

The house seemed strange without Harry. I always looked for him when I came home. I wondered if I'd done the right thing, sending him off. This was time we could be spending with him...but Harry wanted to go. That was what mattered. They were his family, too. Whether he thought he was seeing them for the last time, I don't know.

He called several times while he was away. The kids were anxious to talk to Daddy. He sounded tired, but was enjoying his many visits.

I'd sent Harry to New York with mostly sweatpants and sweatshirts, as they were warm, pulled on easily, and fit him nicely. They discreetly covered the thin, frail body hidden underneath. I'd tried many times to buy him new jeans, but he flatly refused. He kept insisting he had plenty of clothes waiting for him, when he gained his weight back.

While there, he contacted Bert and Keith, our dear friends who share the same wedding anniversary. Keith and Harry had once talked of starting a used car business together. It would have been very successful, I have no doubt. Two smart businessmen, both with a great love and knowledge of automobiles. When Harry stopped by, Bert wasn't home. She later confided she was glad she wasn't. Keith and Harry sat and talked for a couple of hours. It must have been difficult for Keith to see him in that condition, tired and weak, weighing about one hundred twenty pounds.

Keith told me they had a wonderful visit, talking cars, laughing over old times. He also said Harry mentioned starting some sort of automotive business, when he got better.

Harry also visited Bob and Claudia. They told me, later on, they were shocked at his appearance. This was especially true for Claudia, who had just seen him in August. His color and his *eyes,* she said. Not only the dark circles beneath them, but they were glassy. They stared back at her, several times, almost looking through her. She also told me Harry seemed almost tranquilized at times. Claudia had made a big dinner and thought he ate well. They sat and visited a few hours afterwards, small talk, but no mention of his illness. Strangely, Harry thanked Claudia for being my friend. He told her he didn't know what I would do without her friendship. While the comment was true, it was an odd thing for Harry to say. He wasn't an emotional type of guy, especially with his friends.

When they said good-bye at the door, both Bob and Claudia knew this really was their last farewell. Unable to bear this, Claudia called Harry the next day, to ask if they could squeeze one more get together in before he went back. "No," Harry had said, "I'm sorry, I won't be able to. But we did have a nice visit."

A strange coincidence occurred while he was away. With so much housework put on hold, I had arranged for a day off. While busy straightening up, the phone rang. It was Sal, an old friend of Harry's, a former coworker from Long Island. Although they hadn't worked together in many years, they still kept in touch by phone every so often. Harry had told him about his cancer, but apparently not the seriousness of it. Sal was amazed to hear Harry was in Long Island. I gave him Harry's parents' phone number and told him I was sure Harry would love to hear from him.

Later that afternoon, Sal called again. "You won't believe this," he excitedly began. "Less than an hour after I called you,

Harry walked into my office. I hadn't gotten a chance to call his folks yet. He just stopped by!" Sal told me they went for lunch at a nearby bar and caught up on the latest news. Harry didn't order any food and barely sipped at his one and only beer. I asked if Harry had mentioned his illness. Sal said Harry mentioned he was still undergoing chemotherapy treatments, but that was all.

"He's real sick, Sal," I sadly told him. "The treatments haven't worked so far."

"I know Wendy... he's so...thin." I thanked him again, for his thoughtful phone call, and we said our good-byes. Every so often, to this day, Sal calls me to see how we're all doing.

Once again, I wondered what was going on in Harry's mind.

The night before Harry was to come home, I called to speak to him. Since he wasn't home, Peggy and I talked briefly. I was concerned about Harry's condition. She told me he was eating better, which I was relieved to hear. She asked me if I knew he was still smoking. Again, I was shocked. He hadn't hidden his smoking from his mother, either. Before I could answer, she asked, "How could you let him smoke?"

"I'm not *letting* him smoke," I tried to explain. "I have tried to stop him. There was nothing I could do." I know she was very upset about it. We all were.

Harry's last day on Long Island was spent at his sister's house. There was a huge family gathering for his younger sister's birthday. Several of his aunts, uncles and cousins were there, which was wonderful for Harry, as well. I'm sure it was an emotional, but special, memory for them all.

Sunday night, Nov.10th, the kids and I went to pick up their father at the airport. They had made "Welcome Home, Daddy" signs, which they excitedly displayed. Harry came down the ramp, looking weary but happy. He walked slowly but steadily, gradually giving us all kisses and hugs. Coming back, he had checked in his carry-on bag. Although it was small and light, he claimed it was too heavy for him to carry. It was late, and we all went to bed once we arrived home.

Monday morning was a holiday, Veterans Day. The banks were closed, so I had a much appreciated day off. I was still in bed, when Harry was getting dressed. Standing in his underwear, I was startled at the sight. The band on his underpants' leg exposed a huge gap, hanging inches away from his legs. They had become so thin, the underwear that once snugged his thighs tightly, now hung freely. His body was so bony, it was skeletal-like. He looked as though he were starving to death.

As I looked up, I noticed the bicep on his left arm was grossly swollen, almost twice the size of the other. "Harry," I asked cautiously, "what happened to *your arm*?"

He looked in the mirror, then flopped down on the edge of the bed. "*Oh God,*" he let out with a deep sigh, "*What now*?"

Harry was scheduled to see Dr. Deligdish that afternoon. I offered to go along, but he didn't want me to. He was going to receive his first dosage of the new chemo treatment, which could take a few hours. He told me he'd be fine and if he needed me, he would call. Once outside, his car wouldn't start. In a hurry, he yelled in the door to tell me he was taking my car, and that he would mess with his later.

Several hours went by. Since I didn't hear from him, I assumed his chemotherapy treatment had held him up. The kids asked when he would be coming home, several times. By four o'clock in the afternoon, however, I began to get concerned. I called the doctor's office and asked to speak to Harry. The nurse was surprised I didn't know where he was. "Harry's at the hospital," she said, "getting a CAT-scan of his arm. We thought he called you."

I hung up the phone, confused but also very worried. I desperately wanted to be with him. I called to the kids and told them I was going to see their father and I'd be back shortly. As I ran out the door, I realized I had no car to drive! Frantic, I hurried next door and asked my neighbor, Bill, if he'd drop me off at the hospital. I quickly explained as we took off. Although I told him I would be fine if he just left me at the entrance, he insisted on coming in with me.

We inquired at the front desk and were told Harry had been released, fifteen minutes earlier. I stood there, both baffled and distressed. I asked if it would be possible for me to call my husband's doctor on her phone. Graciously, the receptionist dialed the number for me. I was bewildered and wanted to hear from Deligdish just what was going on.

The doctor got on the phone immediately. He explained he was concerned about the swelling in Harry's arm and suspected it was a new tumor, cutting off the circulation in that area. A CAT-scan had been ordered to confirm his suspicions. Dr. Deligdish also mentioned, due to the fact Harry's white blood cell count was now very high, (50,000) he hadn't been able to start his new chemotherapy that day. Instead, they scheduled him for a blood transfusion on Wednesday and the chemo was rescheduled for Friday.

I listened intently, trying to read between the lines. "Why is this all happening?"

"We'll know more when I get the scan results back," he told me, "but my biggest concern is to get his blood cell count back down. It's dangerously high. I had a serious talk with Harry. I told him he should be spending quality time with his family and that he should get his affairs in order. I also mentioned that, although we're doing everything possible to help him, his cancer seems to be very difficult to treat. I told him that at this time, his prognosis was not good."

"You told him *that*?," I gasped. "What did he say?"

"He didn't say much really. He wanted to know when we would be able to start the new treatment."

I thanked him for his help and Bill and I left.

On the way home,Bill wanted to know what the doctor had said. I told him about the new tumor, but left the rest out. Except for some soft music in the background, we drove home in silence.

Chapter 20

Nov. 12

Tuesday morning, Harry was already up and in the kitchen when my alarm went off. He hadn't slept much the night before. I'd been aware of his tossing and turning, desperately trying to get comfortable. I was exhausted, but, felt worse for him. His pain and suffering were an open book now. There was nothing I could do to help.

I went to work and called home several times. Harry spent the day in bed, which probably contributed to him not being able to sleep at night. That evening, he refused to eat. I talked him into a small amount of the Ensure, to which I added an egg and chocolate ice cream. He spent the night wandering back and forth, between the bedroom and the den couch. Harry's low grade fevers were constant now. He was always cold and shivering.

I hurried the kids to bed, as I felt Harry really needed some peace and quiet. We watched TV in bed for a while, then went to sleep. There was not much said between us, but the house was calm and serene.

Nov. 13

Early Wednesday morning, I again found Harry at the kitchen table. Neither one of us had slept much at all. I was beginning to feel like a zombie, functioning at home and work much like a robot. Harry mentioned he was having his blood transfusion that day. I asked if he needed me to be there, but again, the answer was no. I hugged him good-bye and left.

I wanted to tell him how sorry I was. How bad I felt. How I wished with all my heart that I could make this all go away. But I had written all that in the letter, so I knew there wasn't much more I could say.

Harry spent most of the day at Deligdish's office. They were able to do the transfusion there. He read several magazines and tried to sleep. It must have seemed like an eternity. One by one, friends had begun to go down to the local blood bank and donate blood. Gail and George, girls at work and their husbands. Everyone knew Harry needed blood. What we didn't know was, the minute this fresh, wholesome blood entered his veins, the white blood cells consumed the red blood cells immediately. The cancer had now taken over. Harry was no longer in control of his body. Not even Dr. Deligdish's transfusions could help now.

That night, while Harry was tossing and turning, I could hear soft, quiet moans. I called his name but he was asleep. I got up and went into the guest bed. I slept a little, but probably not much better. I was endlessly consumed with thoughts. My *heart* still wanted to believe that somehow, some where, this madness would stop. But my *brain* would tell me that Harry was dying, and there was not a thing anyone could do. My emotions were playing tug of war and I knew which side was winning.

Nov. 14

On Thursday morning, as I sleepily poured milk into my bowl, Harry came out of our room. "Where were you last night?" he somberly asked.

Surprised he'd even realized I was gone, I answered, "I thought you'd sleep better if you had the whole bed to yourself,

Harry. I know you're having a really hard time at night."

Looking at me sadly, he said, "Please don't leave me there alone. I hate waking up and not having you there. I know I'm probably keeping you up half the night, but please don't leave again. I really want you there."

I was shocked. I went over and hugged him. I told him how sorry I was, and that I would *never* do that again.

How selfish could I be? If Harry wanted me by his side, then *no matter what*, that's where I would be.

That afternoon, Harry tried to mow the lawn. Bill, from next door, noticed him struggling with the grass catcher and came over to help. Harry was no longer able to lift off the bag. How incompetent that must have made him feel. Here he was, depending on a man almost twice his age, to do such a simple task. He mowed about half the yard, then put the mower away and went in to rest. Bill also mentioned that later on that same day, Harry had gotten on his bicycle and tried to ride down the street. His balance was off, so he wobbled along until he almost fell over. What possessed him to take that bike out then? He hadn't ridden it in months. I can only assume he was determined to build up his declining strength, any possible way he could.

Again Harry ate practically nothing for dinner. I began to notice his motions were slower, more deliberate. His breathing had become shallow. I knew he was very, very tired.

Nov. 15

Friday finally came. The long awaited weekend was almost here. Harry drove me to work. He'd hired a man to do some work on his car, which still wasn't running right. In almost sixteen years of marriage, this was one of the rare times someone else was working on one of Harry's cars. But it wasn't physically possible for him to do the work anymore and he knew it. Harry's limitations were real to him now.

Harry drove himself to receive the long awaited new chemo

treatment. Again, he was able to receive this type at the doctor's office. Although his white blood-cell counts hadn't improved, they gave him the chemo treatment anyway. The blood transfusion hadn't helped. Harry's cancer was running rampant. Now, more than ever, the chemotherapy was necessary. It was a final, last hope.

Harry spent the entire day there.

I got off work at 6:15 on Friday evening. Harry was waiting for me in the car, out front. He'd just picked up the girls at a friend's home, nearby. Kathy, from work, came out with me and went over to our car. She wanted to invite us to a surprise birthday party for her husband, the following evening. Harry shook his head and told her he didn't think so, but if he felt better, we'd be there.

I got in the car; within minutes, I knew something was wrong. Harry's driving was erratic. It was unusually slow, and several times, he drove up onto the curb a bit. His speech was also somewhat slurred. If I didn't know better, I'd have thought he was drunk. His eyes even gave off that glassy, hazy look. I was scared to death, but said nothing. Luckily, we arrived home safely.

There was a note from Chris. He and a friend had gone to the local bowling alley. They needed to be picked up at nine o'clock. We ordered pizza, Harry ate a small slice, and I began straightening up. A little before nine, Harry offered to go pick up the boys. Since he seemed somewhat better, I decided it would be all right.

When I think back on this, I wonder how I could possibly have let him go. I certainly knew something was wrong, but I didn't know exactly what. My only excuse is that I knew I couldn't bring myself to tell him he wasn't capable of driving. Harry was such a proud, independent man. Was it coming to that?

God watched over Harry and the kids that night, because

everything went all right. He picked them up, stopped for gas and a lottery ticket, and drove the other boy home. Chris and his Dad arrived back home safely around 9:30. Thankfully, there hadn't been much traffic that night. None of us knew it then, but Harry had driven for the last time.

Chapter 21

Nov. 16

When I woke up on Saturday morning, Harry wasn't in our bed. I searched for him, from room to room. I finally found him, sitting quite oddly on the guest room bed. He was barely on the edge, staring mindlessly ahead at the bare wall. I watched him for a moment, before I asked him what he was doing. He slowly turned toward me, his face contorted in a state of confusion. "Have you found it yet?" he suddenly asked.

"Found what?" I wondered.

He didn't answer me, just continued his fixation on the bedroom wall. I walked over to Harry and sat beside him. I asked him if he had slept at all that night but, once again, there was no reply.

Gradually, I coaxed Harry back to our room and helped him back to bed. Although I was quite concerned with his odd behavior, I justified his delirium as lack of sleep. I knew he was exhausted. Within minutes I returned, only to find him sitting up, again on the edge of the bed. His back was as erect as an arrow, his eyes again gazing at the wall. He began to point to the light switch and mumble some sort of incoherent words. Not knowing exactly what he was saying, I assumed he wanted the light on. I turned it on, but he shook his head, as if to say he wanted it off. This went on for several minutes, before I finally told him to forget the light, that he needed to go back to sleep. I knew he just needed to get some rest.

A short while later, my father drove up. He'd come for the weekend and was anxious to show us the new car he'd just purchased. I hastily caught him at the front door and explained what had been going on that morning. He went into our room, came out a few minutes later, and told me he also didn't understand anything Harry was saying. What in the world was wrong?

I managed to keep Harry in our room most of the morning. He didn't sleep at all. Instead, he would sit up and say things, walk around a bit, then lie back down. On one trip to the bathroom, he decided to cut his toenails, but couldn't figure out how the clippers worked. Later on, I found both our toothbrushes soaking in a cup of soapy water.

Fortunately, the kids slept late that day. Chris was the only one who came into our room to see his Dad, later in the morning. After a few moments, he came out and asked me what was wrong with Daddy. "He's talking kind of crazy," he said.

I tried to explain, which was difficult, because I really didn't know myself. The girls never did come into our room that day. I can only assume they thought he was sleeping. The door was closed; and at this point, that had become normal to them.

By early afternoon, when there was no improvement, I decided to call Dr. Deligdish. I went into the guest room, to talk privately. The answering service told me the doctor would call right back. He did, and listened to me with deep concentration. He told me there were several possibilities as to what was causing Harry's confusion. More than likely, it was from lack of oxygen in his blood, a result of his high white blood cell count. He felt another blood transfusion might be necessary. Also, the cancer could have traveled to his brain. Since lung cancer very commonly invades the brain as well, the doctor felt another CAT-scan might be in order.

Dear God, what next?

"Do you want to bring him in, or do you want to wait and see if his condition improves?" he asked. "If you don't think you can handle this, we can admit him," he added.

I thought about it for a minute. No, I wanted to take care of him myself. It was the weekend, I was home, my father was there. "No, I'll be all right," I answered. "I'll keep him home. Harry hates the hospital, so I really don't want to do that to him." We were just about to hang up, when I blurted out, "Dr. Deligdish, please tell me, is Harry... *dying?"* I had to know.

His voice was soft and comforting. "Yes, Wendy. It appears so. You need to get...prepared."

Prepared? How does one *prepare* for that? "How long do you think he has? Weeks...months?", I cautiously asked.

He thought for a moment, then answered, "Weeks, maybe. I really don't know. It's hard to say. If we can get his white blood cell count in order, then perhaps the new chemotherapy might be able to buy him some more time...Maybe."

For some strange reason, I then asked if he thought Harry could make it until Christmas. I just wanted us all to be together one more Christmas. Again, he didn't know. But there was not much conviction in his voice.

Before he hung up, Dr. Deligdish asked me to keep him posted on Harry's condition throughout the day. I sat on the end of the bed, my mind racing in circles. I listened to the kids running about, on the other side of the door, laughing, playing. I *had* to tell them. I had to *prepare* us all.

I spent the rest of the afternoon going back and forth, bringing Harry small snacks, encouraging him to eat or rest. He never did sleep. He had the television on, a football game. But most of what he said was still incoherent.

Later on in the day, I found him in the garage. He had a pair of pliers in his hand, and appeared to be fixing something. It was a small, copper valve that was one solid piece. He was trying to loosen it in the middle, but as I looked at it, I could see that it wasn't possible. I tried to take the tools from him and he got angry. "I can do it!," he snapped. I told him that I knew he could, but he should go in and rest, and try and fix it later.

To this day, my heart goes out to all caregivers of Alzheimer's patients. It is like caring for a child. I caught myself talking to Harry like I would a two year old. Telling him to be good, and go back to bed. How demeaning.

It was sometime after dinner, as I was taking his half-eaten plate of food away, I noticed Harry had taken his socks off. I couldn't believe my eyes. His feet were swollen twice their size. One touch of a finger left a deep, lasting impression.

"Mom, what's wrong with his feet?" Chris asked, as he came in from the kitchen. I just shook my head and announced that I was going to call the doctor.

Dr. Deligdish sounded concerned. "You'd better bring him in," he told me.

I explained I was worried Harry wouldn't cooperate. He'd made it clear he didn't want to go back to that hospital. "Call an ambulance, if necessary," the doctor ordered.

I was frantic. I knew I didn't want to have to do that. I went over to Harry and slowly explained to him the doctor was concerned about his swollen feet, and wanted to see him at the hospital. I wasn't sure what he understood at first, but he suddenly answered, "No!"

I decided to call George. I quickly told him what was going on, and that I might need his brute strength to help me get Harry to the emergency room. George said he would come right over, but I told him I'd call him back if I needed his help.

As I walked into our room, I asked Chris to help me get Daddy dressed. We pulled on a fresh pair of sweatpants, and a clean shirt. It was impossible to attempt his sneakers, so we settled for a pair of slippers that barely squeezed on.

"Harry", I said quietly, "we have to go to the hospital. Dr.

Deligdish wants to check your feet." I held my breath waiting for his response...

"O.K.," he replied, and that was that. I don't know if he surrendered to the idea or if he simply forgot he didn't want to go. Nevertheless, he walked through the kitchen, passed the girls and my father, said good-bye, and got in the car. I quickly explained to everyone where we were going, and why, and off we went.

The emergency crew checked Harry thoroughly. They asked several questions, his name, who was president, etc., all of which he was able to answer correctly, chuckling at the ridiculousness of it all. He did, however, still get his words mixed up when he was trying to speak an entire sentence.

They admitted him about ten o'clock. Dr. Deligdish had ordered a CAT-scan on his brain to be done that evening. They wheeled Harry, to a room, down a long, silent hallway. I was waiting outside when the nurse came for me.

"He keeps asking for you. He wants you to be with him. You're really not supposed to come in, but it's all right, there's no one around." I was deeply moved. Here I hadn't even been sure if Harry knew who I was, and yet he certainly did. He wanted me by his side. He really *didn't* want to go through this alone.

I went in and held his hand, until she slid him into the long, cylinder-like tunnel. It took several minutes before it was done. Harry had to lie very still, which he amazingly did. However, when she was through, he squeezed my hand and thanked me for being there.

Chapter 22

Nov. 17

Even though I had gotten home from the hospital about midnight Saturday night, I got up early Sunday morning. I needed to get some housework done and get back to see Harry. The kids asked if they could come and see Daddy, but I wanted to see how he was doing first. Again, I guess I was trying to protect them.

When I got to the hospital around ten o'clock, Harry was sitting up in bed. He was connected to several tubes, all hanging from IV poles behind him, providing another blood transfusion, as well as glucose water and some sort of antibiotic. His words were clearer but he still seemed distant, and so very tired. I sat with him most of the day, encouraging him to eat, which he barely did.

As we were watching TV, I noticed Harry staring out into the hallway. There hung some abstract paintings, of no real definite form, just bright, bold colors. He began to tell me how he had been studying those "pictures" all day, how pretty he thought they were. He wanted to know what I thought they looked like. I told him I really didn't know, but the colors were nice and bright. He said he thought they looked like animals — rabbits, deer, sheep. He really loved those paintings. Whatever state of mind he was actually in, the artwork seemed to give him some form of serene comfort.

I left after I helped Harry eat some dinner. I'd been there all day. He hadn't slept at all and I knew he had to be tired. The nurse said they would be giving him a sleeping pill that evening. I didn't say so, but I could have used one myself.

I went home and told the kids Daddy was feeling better, and perhaps they could see him the next day, after school. I then called my manager and told her what had gone on, and that I would need the next day off. I felt I needed to be with Harry. I assured her I would be in on Tuesday, then asked her if there were any possible way I could go back on the teller line, work back in the drive-through, away from the immediate public.

In my current position, I sat at the first desk, where the customers first entered the lobby. It was hard to be cheerful and relaxed, with all that was going on in my life. I'm certain I wasn't a vision of gloom, but it was no longer easy to pretend nothing was wrong. My manager sympathized, but explained that, unfortunately, it wasn't possible. It wouldn't be *fair* to everyone else. She suggested that I take a leave of absence from work and offered to check into the procedure for me. I thanked her, but knew that wasn't an option. A family leave was unpaid, and even as small as my salary was, we needed every penny of it.

Even at the time, I knew this treatment of my situation was not my manager's fault. She was a wonderful, caring boss, and I knew she would do anything she could do, to help me. It was just not bank policy and procedure, however, to consider their employees' home-life problems. I did understand the unfairness of me asking for "special considerations". However, I knew in my heart, *I* would be more than willing to help a fellow employee out in a similar situation. Although an unpaid leave could be very helpful, I would say in most people's circumstances, it's not feasible.

It is my understanding that the bank now offers all employees, in this type of family-illness situation, help and understanding. Time off with pay is now offered. Fewer hours and smaller workloads. With all my heart, I hope that is true. I also hope I never have to find out.

Nov. 18

Monday morning I did a few loads of wash, then headed for the hospital. I said good-bye to my father, who was headed home for a dentist appointment. He offered to cancel it, but I told him I would be fine; if I needed him back, I would call.

I cannot stress enough, what my father's love and support meant to me. He was my Rock of Gibraltar, on which I frequently leaned.

Once at the hospital, I was amazed to see Harry doing so well. He still seemed restless, but his words were correct and precise once more. We walked up and down the hallway several times, carting along the two IV poles behind us. He would only last a few minutes, before he was tired, but we were still proud of his accomplishment. He ate much better, but still needed my aid. I offered to feed him, and was surprised when he agreed. We chatted, off and on, and although he was quite tired and short of breath, his spirits were good.

Dr. Deligdish stopped by while I was there. He was also pleased with Harry's progress. He told Harry he was scheduled for a shunt to be put in his back the next day, to prepare him for his upcoming chemo treatment. This was a small tube, which would be placed permanently in a vein, making it unnecessary to search for a new IV line each time. Poor Harry's veins had been poked and prodded so many times, they had more or less collapsed. The procedure sounded simple and painless.

Later in the day, Gail, the social worker who ran the cancer support group, came in for visit. She talked for a while, joking with Harry on the task of raising teenagers. This was the first time they had met, as Harry had never gone to any of the meetings. Before she left, Gail asked Harry if he had previously filled out a *Living Will.* This document states that one does not wish to be kept alive by artificial machines, or resuscitated once cardiac arrest has taken place. It is a legal, binding agreement, which hospitals honor and respect. Since Harry hadn't signed one as of yet, she handed him one she had on her clipboard.

Harry sloppily filled it out. Gail and I witnessed his signature. I don't know if this was a planned meeting, or if bringing the document was coincidental. I was a little apprehensive when she brought it up, wondering what Harry was thinking. But Harry had filled it out, with no questions asked, so I said nothing.

Shortly after Gail left, dinner arrived. I helped Harry eat — mashed potatoes, roast beef (his favorite) and a few carrots I managed to sneak in. Generally, he ate well. While he was eating, he suddenly brought up my letter. This was the first time he'd mentioned it since coming back from New York. I was shocked he would think of it at all, especially at that moment. However, it seemed to be important to him that we discuss it.

He told me I was right. That we hadn't seemed to communicate very well lately, it was all his fault, and he wanted to try harder. He said he wanted things between us to be better. I explained I didn't think I was right, or he was wrong, but we both needed to work at simply understanding and respecting each other. He told me how much he loved me and how much he appreciated all my love and help. "I don't know how I would have gotten through all this without you," he gently said. I couldn't believe these expressions of love and kindness were coming from Harry, at such a time.

Tears began to flow down my cheeks. I tried to look away, so he wouldn't see them, but that wasn't possible. Harry was quiet for a moment, then let out a long, drawn out sigh and said, "Oh, when is this all going to be over? When am I *going to get better*?"

I began to sob openly. I put my head on his chest and had a good, long cry. *That*, I couldn't answer.

I decided to go home and get the kids. I knew they were anxious to see their father, and he was doing so much better. Once home, I told them I would take the girls to the hospital with me that night, and Chris and I would go together on Tuesday evening. There was a cancer support group dinner on Tuesday and Chris had agreed to be my date. I would take him with me to the hospital after work, we'd visit a while, then head to our dinner. It was all planned.

The girls had a wonderful visit with their daddy. They got a kick out of helping pull the IV poles, as we walked down the hall. Harry seemed a little more restless than before, but was still sharp and alert. Kate told him all about her field trip that day to the town of "Christmas". She excitedly mentioned she had bought him Indian Arrow Heads, for good luck. They had fun making the bed rise up and down, taking a free ride each time. We stayed until almost nine, but it was then time to leave. I told Harry that Chris and I would be back the following afternoon. We all kissed and hugged and said our good-byes.

As we stepped outside, we saw Dr. Deligdish down the hall. We talked about how well Harry was doing. He told me that if Harry continued to improve, he would release him to go home on Thursday. Once home, he suggested I receive some help in caring for Harry. I agreed. He said he would have the local *hospice* group get in touch with me. This is an organization of well-trained people who help with the care of a terminally ill patient. They come to your home and assist not only with the patient's medical needs, but with their emotional needs and the family's as well. They are truly God-sent angels during such desperate times.

I thanked him and we left.

On our way back down the hall, we again passed Harry's room. We all peeked in and waved. Harry was sitting back up again, on the edge of the bed. He smiled and waved back to us. He looked so calm, so composed, *so peaceful.*

As we got into the car, I knew I needed to explain to the kids, the seriousness of Harry's condition. Although he seemed so much better, I felt I should prepare them for what *might happen*, even if it was weeks or months away.

I don't know how I found the words, but I gently explained what was taking place. How the cancer seemed to be spreading, and the chemo treatments hadn't seemed to work. We did talk about the new treatment, and how we hoped it would help. I then stated firmly but lovingly, they needed to understand that Daddy might not get better. *Daddy might die*.

I couldn't believe those words really came from me, but they did. What a horrible, cruel thing to say to these two innocent, little girls. It *was* unfair, but it had to be said.

When we got home, Chris was already in bed, asleep. My first thoughts were to go and wake him and talk to him, too, but I decided to let him sleep. I knew I would have time the next day, either before or after our visit with Harry.

The girls and I cried a lot that night. They asked if they could sleep with me. I held them both in my arms, all night long. There was little I could do to comfort them. I heard soft whimpers well into the night, which gradually gave way to a cold, dark silence.

Chapter 23

Nov. 19

At 6:45 Tuesday morning, my alarm went off as usual. I hopped in the shower, exhausted, but ready to start my day. I had just stepped out, my towel was still draped across me, when the phone rang.

"Is this Wendy Kirchner?" the caller wanted to know. Puzzled, I answered that it was. "This is Holmes Regional Hospital calling. Dr. Deligdish wanted me to call you. He felt you needed to get a good night's sleep, so he asked that I wait until this morning, but we need you to come in right away. Harry slipped into a coma during the night. He's not doing well. It's...only a matter of time."

I paused a few moments, trying to grasp what she had just told me. It didn't make any sense. "But, he was doing so well," I somehow stammered out. "He's in a coma?" "But, people come out of comas, don't they?"

She quickly, but gently replied, "Not this kind...You really need to come...*right away.*"

I hung up the phone and tried to think of what I should do first. There must be a small part of your brain, in your subconscious, that just takes over when you are in a state of shock. I have no idea how I functioned. I know I was trembling terribly. I grabbed the quickest outfit I could find, a pair of jeans, still hanging over a chair, and a cotton T-shirt. I ran a brush through my hair and started to head out my door.

I could hear the girls in the kitchen, bowls and spoons clanking, soft chatter in the background. Chris had already left for his bus. I stopped short and sat on the edge of my bed, realizing I had to make a serious decision. In what probably amounted to a mere sixty seconds, I decided who *would* and who *wouldn't* come along with me that day. I knew this was an extremely important judgment call that ultimately could affect my children's lives forever. Fortunately, I do believe I somehow, some way, made the right one.

I quickly called my father. I blurted out what the nurse had told me and asked him to meet me at the hospital. This poor seventy eight year old man had to scramble around like I was, gathering clothes as he gathered his thoughts. I know this must have been equally difficult for him.

I then called work, fortunate enough to reach one of the early arrivers. She was both sympathetic and supportive and told me we were all in her prayers.

I was desperate to be calm and collected as I entered the girls' room. They were busy getting together books and papers. I told them I was going to the hospital to see Daddy, instead of going to work. I explained he had gone into a coma, during the night, and the doctor wanted me to be there. Ironically, they both knew all about comas.

A young boy from their school had been hit by a car a few weeks before and had been in a coma for a few days. He did come out of it, however, and was expected to make a complete recovery. I guess that's why none of us got panicky when we heard *coma.* Lots of people recover from them. Harry's coma was *different*, however, brought about by totally different circumstances.

Kerin was quiet. She observed my every move, discreetly watching my expression for any clue to my thoughts and feelings. Kate made a comment about how the boy they knew had come out of his coma and was getting better. I gently explained that I needed to get to the hospital to see how Daddy was doing, to see if the doctors were able to help him. I told them there was nothing that they could do, they would have to go to school, but I would be there in the afternoon to pick them up. They didn't protest, fortunately. I guess, deep down, they understood more than I'll ever know.

After dropping the girls off, I turned around and headed for Chris' junior high. It was the opposite direction of the hospital, and I wanted to get there immediately, but, I *knew* I had to get Chris first. Chris needed to be there. For himself, for Harry. And perhaps, most of all, I *needed* Chris there, for me.

As I entered the office, the secretary stood and saw streams of tears pouring down my cheeks. "I need to check my son, Chris Kirchner, out of school. His Dad is in a coma....he's *dying*. I need my son, *now*..."

She immediately had him paged. As Chris turned the corner and saw me, he knew. He put his arm around me and said, "It's O.K., Mom. Don't worry, it's going to be O.K."

We sat down by the edge of Harry's bed, side by side. Chris held my hand, as well as his father's. Harry's eyes were open, but didn't focus on us, or anything else. They wandered, searching the room, exploring every wall and structure, but stopping at nothing. His body continuously twitched and turned. Every so often, his face would twist and contort, looking painful and uncomfortable. It was hard to watch.

My father arrived shortly thereafter. We hugged for a long time. He let out a long, deep breath, shook his head, and sat beside me.

As much as I didn't want to leave, I had to call Harry's family. I knew they would need to make arrangements to come to Florida quickly. I let his parents' phone ring several times. There was no answer. I called again. Still no answer. I could not imagine where they could be! I later learned they were all sleeping so soundly, no one heard the phone. After a failed third attempt, I was desperate. I called Harry's sister, Joan. I could barely get the words out. I told her they all needed to come as soon as possible. She sobbed, as she told me she would call the rest of the family. We tried to comfort each other, but that was not possible. We were all losing Harry and *we all loved him.*

I went back to the room and sat down by Harry's side, getting as close as I could. Chris again took my hand. We all tried to talk to Harry, comfort him, stroke his hands and face. Harry continued to thrust about, more frequently as time went on.

Dr. Deligdish came in around noon, looking distraught. I wanted to know what was going on, why this had happened. "He was doing so great," I repeated.

He explained the CAT-scan on Harry's brain had come back normal, but his white blood cell count had gone so high, there was virtually no oxygen left in his blood. As quick as he received new blood, the cancer ravaged through and took over. It was causing mini strokes, thus the coma and the twisting and turning. I asked if there was any way he could possibly come out of this. I guess I *still* had a small hope, that this, too, would pass. Dr. Deligdish sadly explained he would not, and that even if he *could* come out of it, there would be an extreme amount of brain damage.

That was it. The last spark of hope flickered out. It was over. I longed to hear Harry's voice say my name, but it was at that moment, I knew that would never happen again.

Dr. Deligdish ordered some sort of pain-killer/tranquilizer, and the contortions and restlessness seemed to subside. Harry was much quieter now, taking short, quick breaths through the oxygen mask. Chris, my father and I sat there, speaking to each other only occasionally. My father asked if I wanted to go get some coffee, but I didn't dare leave Harry's side. Chris and his grandfather left briefly, got a drink and a small bite to eat and hurried back.

I watched my husband lie there. He looked so small in the bed. His body seemed that of a small child. How could this be happening...to Harry, to me, to my children? This sort of thing doesn't happen to people you know, let alone to you. This bad movie was real life and it had slowly snuck its way into mine.

Chris came back, while my father went to make some calls. There were so many people to phone. So many people to tell what was going on. He phoned my brother, Wayne, in California. He was shocked. He promised he would be on the next flight out. I'm sure he couldn't get to Florida fast enough. My father tried several times to reach my brother, Warren, in Colorado, but to no avail. He'd apparently just left for a two week camping trip. I had talked to him a few weeks before and told him Harry was awaiting his new treatment. Warren had no way of knowing Harry would take a turn for the worse, so quickly. None of us did.

I called Gail. She didn't know what to say. She was so sad. She just kept repeating this couldn't be happening. I quickly called Claudia at work. We both cried. She was suffering a loss also. She vowed to hang up and make arrangements to catch the next plane from New York.

I went back to Harry's room. There was no change. I watched Chris softly talk to his father. What an unimaginable void there would be in his life.

Gail came up to the room about two o'clock. She'd left work, too upset to stay. She wanted to come by to give her love and support. It was abundant in the room that day.

We all sat by Harry's side, one by one, holding his hands, and each others. Chris kept his arm around me, gently rubbing my shoulders. This fourteen year old boy had to be a man that day. As hard as that task would be, he managed to handle it with such maturity and sophistication, his father would have been proud.

At 2:30, a nurse came in and said that Harry's lungs needed

to be suctioned and they would then move him to a new room, down the hall. I was confused, but was told the doctor wanted us to have more privacy. We waited in the lounge, until a nurse burst into the room to get us. "Harry has gone into cardiac arrest," she blurted out. "You need to come — *right away.*" We all scrambled down the corridor. I could feel my legs quivering. I held Chris' hand tightly.

We walked into the new room. The silence was deafening. Harry had been disconnected from all machines. He was quiet, very still. His chest slowly moved up and down, as we all stood by. He took a final, short, quick breath, and stopped...It was 2:45 p.m.

Harry's struggle was over...

Cigarettes had claimed yet another victim...

Harry was gone.

Epilogue

Shortly after Harry's death, I received a letter from Dr. Deligdish. Thinking it was another bill, I tossed it aside. When I noticed the different type. of envelope, however, I opened it and began to read. I had to sit down. I've printed the letter in its entirety, as I am so deeply moved by its contents. I was later informed this was not usual procedure. The doctor was truly saddened by Harry's passing.

Not that all his patients aren't important to him, by any means. But Harry must have hit a special nerve. Perhaps, because they were so close in age. Maybe Harry's belief and confidence that Dr. Deligdish could save him. Or, just Harry's sweet, uncompromising demeanor. For whatever reason it was written, this letter meant the world to me. He was not just a patient with a number. He was real and his life had real meaning.

I continue to work in the same bank, part time. My children and their many activities have kept me both busy and fulfilled. The writing of this book has certainly occupied a great deal of my time and contributed in my healing as well. What started out as a journal, slowly, over time, became this account of what one family went through living with, day after day, the deadly effects of lung cancer.

At times, this book was difficult to write. Not only did it bring up emotions I had long since buried, but in the midst of it

CRAIG DELIGDISH, M.D.
Diplomate, American Board of Internal Medicine
Diplomate in the Subspecialty of Medical Oncology
Diplomate in the Subspecialty of Hematology

HEMATOLOGY
MEDICAL ONCOLOGY
INTERNAL MEDICINE

November 21, 1991

Mrs. Wendy Kirchner
2486 Nobility Avenue
Melbourne, Florida 32934

Dear Wendy:

Firstly, I would like to express my condolences regarding Harry's passing.

Although medicine has come a long way in the last several decades, there remain several diseases which are extremely difficult to treat. Metastatic lung cancer, is unfortunately, one such disease. Although it initially appeared that the combination of chemotherapy, radiation therapy, and surgery might have successfully eradicated Harry's cancer, this was also unfortunately not the case.

Harry's situation was certainly quite unusual in that his cancer progressed at an alarming rate. He had a very aggressive disease, which did not respond very well to our treatment. Harry was however, in some ways fortunate, in that I believe he was spared the pain which is generally associated with terminal cancer. He was also fortunate to have such a loving and supportive family who was at his side in his hour of need.

I am certain that the last several months have been extremely difficult for you. I am hopeful that the support groups have been of some help, and I only wish that Harry had participated in the support group with you. Cancer is certainly a devastating disease, but it is even more devastating when it affects young people, especially those with families. I know that the next several months and probably the next several years will continue to be difficult for you and your family. If there is anything that I can do to make things easier, please do not hesitate to contact me.

Once again, I would like to express my condolences, as well as those of my wife and all of those in my office who had the pleasure of knowing your husband. If at any time we can be of assistance, I hope you will not hesitate to call on us.

Sincerely,

Craig Deligdish

Craig Deligdish, M.D.

1341 S. HICKORY ST., SUITE 116, MELBOURNE, FL 32901 • (407) 727-3495 all, my father suddenly passed away. He had been so supportive and encouraging, and yet, for a long while afterwards, I lost my enthusiasm to continue. Eventually, as with so many other things, the desire to tell Harry's story returned. To make believers out of smokers. To get the message out about how dangerous and deadly smoking *really is.* And to campaign fiercely against the tobacco companies and cigarette smoking.

Yes, I am angry. Why shouldn't I be? Cigarettes took away my family's hopes and dreams.

They say that something good seems to come of something bad. Yet I certainly had to look long and hard to find the good in this of life's lessons. But as time went on, things had a way of surfacing.

We have all learned that, although life is good, it's not always fair. Bad things do happen to good people. But if you have good health, and a kind, loving family, you have all the riches in the world. Nothing else matters.

Our loss of Harry is still felt every day, but time has promoted healing. It is indeed sad he is gone, then again, he has three children. And so, in each of them, Harry lives on.

Christopher is now a handsome, young man, who towers over me at 6'2"! His passion, repairing and rebuilding car engines, is much like his father's. He recently told me he feels close to his dad, when his head is under the hood of a car.

His present goals are to marry his high school sweetheart, Sarah, and to join the Air Force.

I know Harry is proud of his son and his accomplishments.

Kerin has blossomed into a lovely, beautiful young woman. She is involved in drama, participating in the high school plays. She has the voice of an angel, and her father's great sense of humor. For a while, Kerin played softball. Harry had played for years and I believe this was also a "bond" to her father. After a while, however, she realized soccer was more suitable for her. Through sheer determination, she manages to use all the muscle and power in her petite body and successfully compete. She also volunteers at the local hospital in the pediatric ward.With a career lying in either the medical or drama field, I tell her not to worry. There is an entire world of choices before her.

I'm certain that one "angel" amidst her assorted collection, consists of her loving, proud father, watching over her.

Kate has done the most growing, both physically and emotionally since losing her Dad at age eight. Now a sweet, pretty adolescent, Kate has a deep sensitivity to both people and their situations. A few years ago, her basketball coach was killed in a motorcycle accident. "I feel so sorry for his kids," she said. "I know how they feel."

Her avid pastimes range from piano to basketball and softball! Her athletic abilities most definitely come from Harry, certainly not from me! When she was nine, she hit her first home run. I sat quietly, alone in the stands, and softly cried the rest of the game. Hundreds of ball games later, I cheer her accomplishments proudly. The deep pain has been replaced with peace of mind, knowing that Harry would not want us to continue to grieve. Instead, he would want us to carry on with our life as a family, and remember him always, with love.

Kate has talked of being a psychologist or entering the aerospace field. Whatever her choice, I know both her perseverance and her father's proud and gentle, guiding soul will see her through.

I must state emphatically that our journey from Harry's death until now has not been an easy one. There were many bumpy roads along the way. Whereas anger and turmoil tend to be prevalent in a home full of teenagers, there came a time when I realized our family's tragedy had begin to surface in many difficult forms. We all needed help, I just could not provide.

I searched out a family counseling center. I also want to stress how valuable therapy can be, both during and after a crisis of any sort.

How I found our therapist is a strange coincidence, or,

maybe not. While setting up our first appointment, the pleasant secretary told me she had assigned us a very caring and understanding counselor, named Harry Hillmer. *Harry!* That was too bizarre. I just couldn't do that to my family or to myself. I tried to explain. She was quite kind and compassionate and changed our meeting to be with another man.

At work, later that day, a friend Arlene, listened intently, as I told her the "eerie" Harry story. Suddenly, she grabbed my arm and cried out, "Wendy, call them back! It's a sign. A sign from God! I have a deep feeling about this!" I was half in shock, but she was so emphatic I went to the phone and changed our appointment back to "Harry".

Arlene's premeditated awareness couldn't have been more on target. Harry Hillmer, our therapist, turned out to be an angel sent to us after all. Using our own tools and skills, he helped us all grieve, forgive and heal.

Thank you God, for sending us — *our other Harry.*

In doing my research for this book, I obtained Harry's medical records from Dr. Deligdish. Whereas, most of the medical jargon was much too complicated for me, I did find some surprising information. One such item was the fact that throughout this medical history folder, Dr. Deligdish referred to Harry as "*an unfortunate gentleman*". *Webster's* dictionary defines unfortunate as: "having or bringing bad luck; unlucky". What a profound choice of words. Certainly, getting lung cancer (or any other cancer for that matter), at the young age of thirty seven, is not only rare, but most definitely, *unfortunate.*

What I also found peculiar, were Harry's answers to some questions at his introductory meeting with the doctor. When asked how many packs per year were smoked, Harry's answer was twenty. Anyone, who was remotely acquainted with Harry, could attest that he was rarely seen without a cigarette in his hand. A more accurate figure would have been twenty packs per week.

Did Harry misunderstand the question? Probably not. Instead, I believe he was, like most smokers, in complete denial of his cigarette addiction and its harmful effects.

Lung cancer is an ugly, unmerciful disease. If life through a crystal ball were possible, and lung cancer was eminent, perhaps then, people would stop smoking, or better yet, never start. Unfortunately, we do not have such a life saving device. We only have the hard, cold facts. The medical knowledge that smoking cigarettes will most definitely shorten one's life, impair the quality of it, or — end it.

People can say Harry was going to die anyway. That we all have to die of something, sometime. Harry said that of Gary. How does that justify the death of a young man of thirty eight? Harry was a healthy, strong human being. It certainly was not his time to die. The nicotine got hold of him, while the tar killed him.

We must get this important message out. Lung cancer is preventable!! Show your yourself and your families that your life is worth keeping. Don't wait until tragedy strikes. Stop smoking now. *It is never too late!*

However, if you happen to be the *unfortunate* one to wind up with this unpredictable disease, fight the good fight. Don't give up. There are success stories. I have personally met lots of them. *Life is worth fighting for.*

Most importantly, don't shut yourself out from your loved ones. Share your joys and your sorrows.

Open that door.

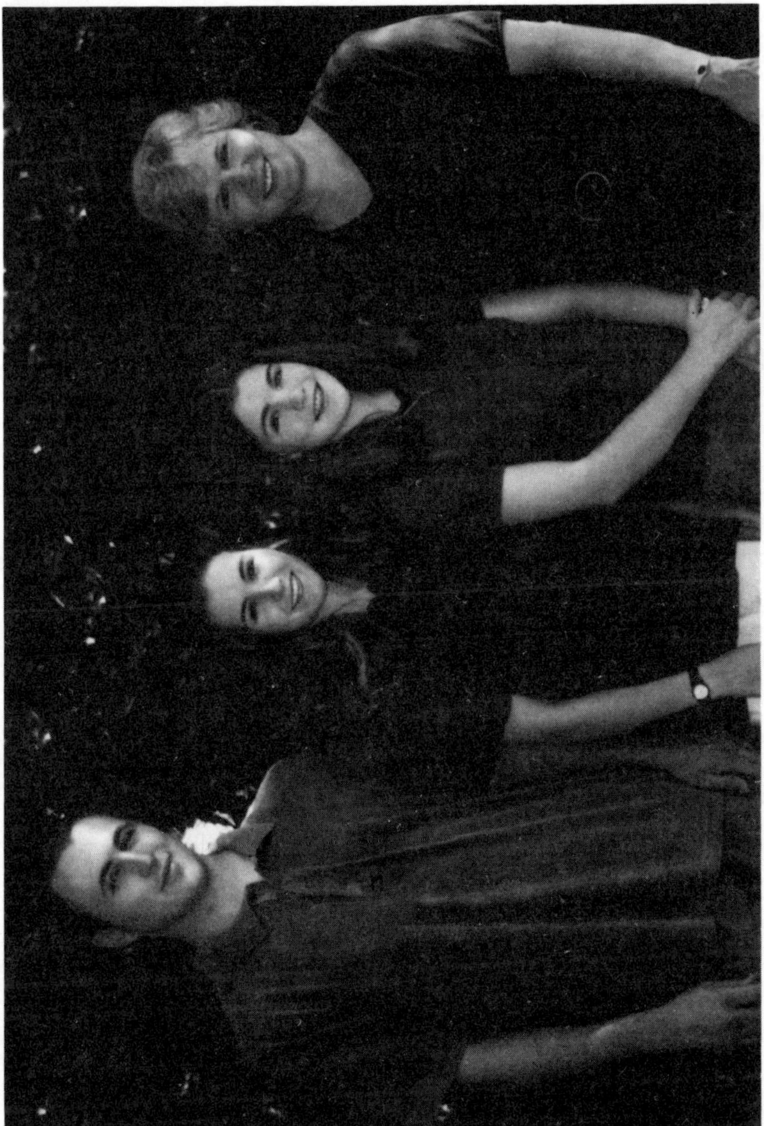

The Kirchners, July 1997 – Chris, Kerin , Kate & Wendy.

Why Quit?

I found the following information during my research of lung cancer and its causes. I discovered many startling facts about tar and nicotine, many hidden by the tobacco companies, which unfortunately, most people don't know.

Cancer is the disease most feared by the majority of people throughout the world. Although cancer has been known and written about throughout history, its widespread prevalence today is no doubt due to the cure of more infectious diseases and the increased life expectancy.

In the United States, there will be approximately 177,000 new cases of lung cancer and 155,000 deaths this year. The average age is sixty years old; it is rare under forty. The five year survival rate is thirteen percent for all stages. Common sites of spread are the brain, liver and bone.

Lung cancer, however, is the most preventable cancer, because its major cause is known — cigarette smoking. The event of the disease is directly related to the continued exposure of its promoting agents. The risk is increased by the number of years an individual has smoked, the number of cigarettes per day, the length of each cigarette, the depth of inhalation and the tar content of cigarettes. The risk of lung cancer decreases when smoking is stopped; after fifteen years, the incidence of lung cancer becomes that of people who have never smoked.

What most people don't know about the tobacco industry, is, in 1969, one tobacco executive admitted his company had increased the level of nicotine in most of their cigarettes. (Tar is what gives cigarette's flavor and causes disease; nicotine is what makes them addictive.) The idea was to "hook" smokers, so the "need to smoke" would be greatly increased. As a result, cigarettes are no longer chopped tobacco leaves rolled in paper. Instead, they are the final product of a refined, intensified, manufacturing process that uses several components from different sources and controls nicotine every step of the way. This practice is not only criminal, but inhumane.

Philip Morris, the leader of tobacco companies, was the first to add ammonia, to heighten the jolt of nicotine, allowing the smoker to get the same buzz from a small amount of the drug. This would assure its cigarettes would provide smokers with a consistent high. Nicotine is an extremely toxic chemical. A sixty-milligram dose is lethal. One cigarette contains approximately a one-milligram impact. Cigarettes, therefore, have been described as a "dirty needle through which the drug nicotine is distributed." Even though the cigarette is the deadliest of everyday products, it remains the least regulated, mostly regarding its ingredients and potency.

Another well kept secret is, in 1980, two scientists, Victor DeNoble and Paul Mele, were hired by Philip Morris to make a safer cigarette, one that would have a less harmful effect on the heart. They succeeded splendidly. They also set up experiments to test the body tolerance to increasingly higher doses of nicotine. These tests were kept top secret. With the use of state of the art laboratory equipment and two hundred rats, DeNoble and Mele not only proved that nicotine was addictive to humans, but was in a class along with heroin and cocaine. Thus, another chemical that promotes dependency. Suddenly, in 1984, they were ordered to stop their research. A few days later, when they came to work, the animals, their logs, everything was gone. Any attempts to publish their results were terminated. As a result, the safer cigarette was forever lost and the nicotine doctoring accelerated.

The most startling fact I found however, was, when it became popular to stop smoking, early in the 60's, the tobacco companies came up with a new ploy. *Low tar and nicotine* cigarettes. How brilliant. Instead of quitting, these cigarettes gave people a workable alternative. However, scientists and the Surgeon General believe these low-yield cigarettes can be a *greater health hazard.*

First of all, the official tar and nicotine ratings are acquired from outdated machines. This equipment extracts one draw of smoke every minute from the cigarette. This was established before cigarettes were filtered. Today, the average smoker's puff rate is one in every thirty-four seconds.

Secondly, most low-tar cigarettes contain tiny holes in their filter that dilute the tar and nicotine coming in. Using the machine, the vents work, but the average person holds the filter with their lips or fingertips. This raises the tar rating as much as *300%*! Also, to make up for the lower doses of tar and nicotine, people tend to puff harder, and longer on these types of cigarettes. This can significantly increase the risk of lung disease. The increased risk is not caused by the number of cigarettes smoked, but rather by how one inhales, disposes, and retains the smoke in their lungs. Worried smokers, therefore, are falsely convinced that lower tar and nicotine cigarettes are safer.

The general public has bought the tobacco companies' bill of goods, allowing them to cash in on the very health fear their product has produced. The sad thing is, their safer, healthier cigarette *is by no means safe at all.*

I learned tobacco smoke contains over 4,000 chemical compounds, including at least 43 different carcinogenic (cancer causing) substances. The 1988 *Surgeon General's Report* concluded that:

• Cigarettes and other forms of tobacco are addicting;

- Nicotine is the drug that causes addiction;
- The pharmacologic and behavioral process which determine tobacco addiction are similar to those which determine addiction to drugs such as heroin and cocaine;
- Nicotine is absorbed readily from tobacco smoke in lungs and is rapidly distributed throughout the body.[1]

How has the tobacco industry gotten away with this for so long? Their vague health-warning label has also provided them protection from product-liability lawsuits. The twenty-five year Federal ban on cigarette advertising also prohibits public service announcements against smoking. Those had previously proven to have considerable impact on the smoking public. Inevitably, the tobacco industry must face the possibility, even the probability, that someday a jury will reach a final verdict against it. Of course, this will mean financial disaster for the cigarette companies. Hopefully, they will be obligated to pay their fair share for the damages their product has inflicted.

Signs and symptoms of lung cancer are: Persistent cough, chest pain, blood or rusty sputum, shortness of breath, hoarseness, weight loss, loss of appetite, recurring fluid in lungs, and anemia.

More people die of lung cancer in one year, than those people who will die from alcohol, AIDS, crack, cocaine, murder and fire — combined. Smoking accounts for about thirty percent of all cancer deaths. Those who smoke two or more packs a day have a mortality rate twelve to twenty five times greater than nonsmokers.

Since 1987, more women have died of lung cancer than breast cancer that, for forty years, was the leading cause of cancer death in women. Lung cancer deaths in 1962 were:[1]

- males - 35,312 females - 6,064

  compared to 1992
- males - 91,405 females - 54,538

About 10% of lung cancer cases occur in people who do not smoke. Work related hazards, air pollution and other environmental factors are involved. Workers who are exposed to cancer–causing substances such as asbestos, face an even greater chance of developing lung cancer if they smoke. 50% of patients with fatal cancer could have been saved, had they used existing knowledge about smoking, diet, exercise and early detection.

The National Cancer Institute studying the cause, prevention, diagnosis, and treatment of lung cancer, found if the number of smokers could be substantially reduced, thousands of lives could be saved. In smokers who stop smoking when precancerous changes are found, damaged lung tissue often returns to normal.

The September, 1990 *Surgeon General* report outlined the benefits of stopping smoking. People who quit smoking, regardless of their age, live longer than people who continue to smoke. Smokers who quit before the age of fifty have half the risk of dying in the next fifteen years, compared with those who continue to smoke. Quitting smoking substantially decreases the risk of lung, laryngeal, esophageal, oral, pancreatic, bladder and cervical cancers. There is also a greater reduction in the risk of other major diseases, such as heart disease and cardiovascular disease.

In a gallop poll among smokers:[1]

- 65% believe their health has already been affected;
- 78% believe that serious health problems are likely if they continue;
- 81% would not start smoking if they could do it over;
- 75% say they are addicted.

Second hand smoke has also become a valid concern. Each year, about 3,000 non-smoking adults die of lung cancer, as a result of breathing the smoke of others' cigarettes. The risk of dying of lung cancer is 30% higher for a non-smoker living with a smoker, compared with a non-smoker living with a non-smoker. Children exposed to second hand smoke have increased risks of respiratory illnesses and infections, impaired development of lung function and middle ear infections. Infants born to women who smoked during pregnancy are more likely to die of Sudden Infant Death Syndrome.

A one year survival rate has risen from 32% in 1973 to 41% in the 90's. A five year survival rate for all stages combined is only 13%. That rate increases to 47% in cases detected when the disease is localized, but only 15% of lung cancers are detected that early.[1]

The long-term survival rate for lung cancer is very low. Recently, however, with better staging techniques and better results from new treatments of chemotherapy, there is hope a cure may be found for individuals who have been in remission.

It is certainly no easy task to quit smoking. Although the addictive drug nicotine makes it quite difficult, it is not impossible. Especially if the will to stop is there. Today there are several choices, compared to the one and only option of "going cold turkey", of years ago. *Nicorette*, the gum, and *Nicoderm*, the patch, (both endorsed by the *American Cancer Society*) are very successful quitting alternatives. (Although they still require a doctor's prescription, a friend recently told me her dentist gave her one. I was so happy to learn these prescriptions can be obtained so easily). Unlike cigarettes, these stop-smoking aids release nicotine slowly into the body, in carefully controlled dosages throughout the day. This helps decrease the intense craving for cigarettes. Quitting smoking makes a difference right away. Noticeable side effects are:

- Food begins to taste and smell better.
- Within minutes your body begins to heal itself of tar and nicotine's nasty effects.
- It also saves you money. A pack-a-day smoker, who pays two dollars per pack, can expect to save more than seven hundred dollars per year.

The bottom line is — when you quit smoking, you reduce your risk of lung cancer, heart disease, stroke, as well as other lung and respiratory diseases.

The best and only way to improve the statistics is — *stop smoking*, if you do smoke, and — *don't start smoking,* if you don't smoke now. You can do it! And may God bless!!!

[1] *Cancer Facts & Figures– 1996 / American Cancer Society*

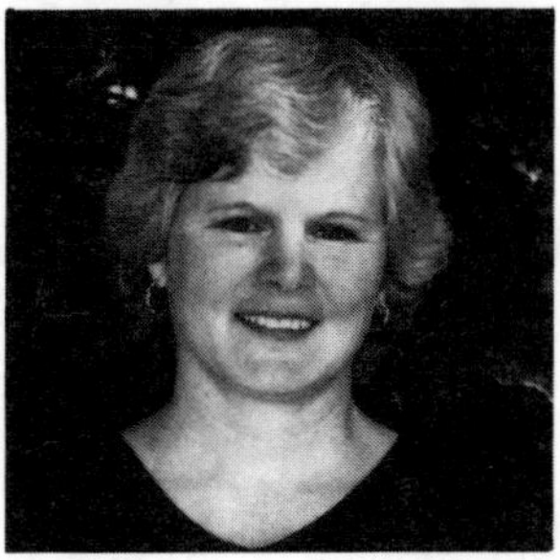

About The Author

Although this is Wendy Kirchner's first published work, she is looking forward to other literary projects in the future.

She continues to live in Melbourne, Florida working "part time in a bank; full time raising her three children." Wendy's dream is to live in a "smoke-free America." She plans to promote her book at anti-smoking and health seminars. Her goal is to encourage people to quit smoking, to convince them that cigarettes really *do* take lives everyday and most importantly, to spread the word that nicotine truly is America's deadliest drug.

It's never too late to quit!!!

To order additional copies of Dying To Smoke,
complete the information below.

Ship to: (please print)

Name ______________________________

Address____________________________

City_______________________________

State____________________Zip________

Area Code (   ) Phone________________

____ of Dying To Smoke @ $9.95ea. $______

Shipping & Handling for first book $ 2.25

Additional books to same address add $1.00ea. ______

Florida residents add 6% ______

Total amount enclosed ______

Make check payable to: **Starr Publishing**

Send to: **Starr Publishing**
P.O. Box 410643
Melbourne, FL 32941-0643

or Call Toll Free: 1-888-259-0005

- -

To order additional copies of Dying To Smoke,
complete the information below.

Ship to: (please print)

Name ______________________________

Address____________________________

City_______________________________

State____________________Zip________

Area Code (   ) Phone________________

____ of Dying To Smoke @ $9.95ea. $______

Shipping & Handling for first book $ 2.25

additional books to same address add $1.00ea. ______

Florida residents add 6% ______

Total amount enclosed ______

Make check payable to: **Starr Publishing**

Send to: **Starr Publishing**
P.O. Box 410643
Melbourne, FL 32941-0643

or Call Toll Free: 1-888-259-0005